FOOD LABELING

Toward National Uniformity

Committee on
State Food Labeling

FOOD AND NUTRITION BOARD
INSTITUTE OF MEDICINE

Donna V. Porter and Robert O. Earl, Editors

NATIONAL ACADEMY PRESS
Washington, D.C. 1992

National Academy Press ● 2101 Constitution Avenue, N.W. ● Washington, D.C. 20418

This study was supported by project no. 282-89-0022 from the Public Health Service, U.S. Department of Health and Human Services.

Library of Congress Catalog Card No. 92-60416

International Standard Book Number 0-309-04737-4

Additional copies of this report are available from:

National Academy Press
2101 Constitution Avenue, N.W.
Washington, DC 20418

S585

Printed in the United States of America

The serpent has been a symbol of long life, healing, and knowledge among almost all cultures and religions since the beginning of recorded history. The image adopted as a logotype by the Institute of Medicine is based on a relief carving from ancient Greece, now held by the Staatlichemuseen in Berlin.

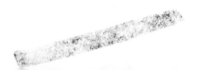

COMMITTEE ON STATE FOOD LABELING

J. PAUL HILE (*Chair*), Phoenix Regulatory Associates, Ltd., Sterling, Virginia

MARY M. HESLIN (*Vice Chair*), Consultant, Hartford, Connecticut

SANDRA O. ARCHIBALD, Food Research Institute, Stanford University, Stanford, California

MARSHA N. COHEN, Hastings College of the Law, University of California, San Francisco, California

JOHN W. ERDMAN, Jr., Department of Food Science and Division of Nutritional Sciences, College of Agriculture, University of Illinois, Urbana, Illinois

JESSE F. GREGORY III, Food Science and Human Nutrition Department, Institute of Food and Agricultural Sciences, University of Florida, Gainesville, Florida

TIMOTHY M. HAMMONDS, Research and Education, Food Marketing Institute, Washington, D.C.

ALVIN J. LORMAN, Akin, Gump, Hauer & Feld, Washington, D.C.

WALTER H. MEYER, Consultant, Cincinnati, Ohio

PATRICIA M. MORRIS, Public Voice for Food and Health Policy, Washington, D.C.

LAURA S. SIMS, College of Human Ecology, University of Maryland, College Park, Maryland

BAILUS WALKER, Jr., College of Public Health, University of Oklahoma Health Sciences Center, Oklahoma City, Oklahoma

NANCY S. WELLMAN, Department of Dietetics and Nutrition, Florida International University, Miami, Florida

Staff

DONNA V. PORTER, Project Director
ROBERT O. EARL, Staff Officer
BARBARA L. MATOS, Project Assistant

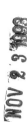

ROY M. PITKIN (*Ex Officio*),† Department of Obstetrics and Gynecology, School of Medicine, University of California, Los Angeles, California

STEVE L. TAYLOR (*Ex Officio*), Department of Food Science and Technology, University of Nebraska, Lincoln, Nebraska

* Member, National Academy of Sciences
† Member, Institute of Medicine

Staff

CATHERINE E. WOTEKI, Director
MARCIA S. LEWIS, Administrative Assistant
SUSAN M. WYATT, Financial Associate

Preface

The Committee on State Food Labeling was assembled in the spring of 1991 by the Food and Nutrition Board (FNB) of the Institute of Medicine (IOM) to conduct a study of selected Federal and State food labeling requirements. The study was initiated in response to the Nutrition Labeling and Education Act of 1990 (NLEA; P.L. 101-535). NLEA preempted all State and local misbranding laws and regulations on a fixed schedule in order to achieve national uniformity. One provision of Section 6 of NLEA required the Secretary of Health and Human Services to enter into a contract with a public or nonprofit private entity to conduct a study of State and local laws that require food labeling of the type mandated by certain misbranding provisions of the Federal Food, Drug, and Cosmetic Act of 1938, as amended (FDCA)—that is, Sections 403(b), 403 (d), 403(f), 403(h), 403(i)(1), and 403(k). The study was also to consider whether the Food and Drug Administration (FDA) has been adequately implementing those sections prior to the effective date of preemption of related State and local requirements.

FDA, the study's sponsoring agency, contracted with IOM based on the Institute's expertise in food labeling issues, which was demonstrated by the 1990 report *Nutrition Labeling: Issues and Directions for the 1990s*. The 13 members of the Committee of State Food Labeling were selected for their expertise in consumer affairs, dietetics, Federal and State food regulatory policy, food law, food production and marketing, food science, human nutrition, and public health.

From the first meeting of the Committee, its members realized that there was a broad array of issues to be explored, some of which were outside their areas of experience. Consequently, the Committee gathered additional needed information through a public meeting, panel discussions at

vii

Committee meetings, requests to the States, and communications with public interest groups, trade associations, and organizations representing food and drug officials. The Committee welcomed information from all outside sources. Further, the Committee recognized that the study was not typical of those regularly conducted by the Institute of Medicine. Beyond an understanding of the food, nutrition, and public health sciences important to the study, there was a need to consider Federal administrative procedures, the policy relationships of different levels of government, the Federal regulatory process, economic issues and consumer concerns. The composition of the Committee established by the Academy was multidisciplinary in nature to meet these diverse needs.

The Committee aggressively pursued collection of the information it identified as necessary to accomplish the requirements of the study outlined in NLEA. The Committee requested the 50 States, selected larger municipalities, and FDA to provide copies of applicable laws, regulations, and other policy statements promulgated in implementing those statutes. The data received from these requests were voluminous; both the amount of individual effort expended and the number of documents exceeded all expectations. The Committee found, however, that there was no single comprehensive data source available for the compilation of relevant Federal, State, and local labeling and related regulatory requirements. As a consequence, the Committee cannot be certain that all relevant materials that might exist were reviewed. With these caveats, the data the Committee collected are perhaps the most extensive available, and have been categorized and analyzed thoroughly. Following completion of the study, the Committee has planned for all the materials collected from States, localities, and other interested parties to be provided to FDA to allow access by all who wish to review them.

The Committee went beyond the strict limits of its charge for several reasons. First, from a practical standpoint, it was difficult and sometimes impossible to separate the existing State and local requirements into six discrete packages to parallel exactly the six FDCA Sections that are the subject of this report. The Committee, therefore, felt it was necessary to review and comment on all State requirements, except those that were obviously not part of the charge—for example, State requirements that were clearly preempted by other provisions of NLEA (e.g., the definition of ice cream). Second, the NLEA language was ambiguous, leaving unanswered questions regarding the scope of the Committee's inquiry and the status of some current State requirements under its automatic preemption requirements. This ambiguity was particularly true for FDCA Section 403(h), dealing with standards of quality and fill. Section 403(h) as enacted, presumes the existence of standards established under FDCA Section 401. Standards of identity established under Section 401, however, are clearly preempted by NLEA. The Committee decided early in its deliberations that such questions of statutory interpretation were beyond its charge.

Finally, a wide variety of views emerged from the information provided to the Committee on the adequacy of FDA's implementation of the six FDCA Sections. In this regard, the Committee decided to review all materials and comments that were submitted and, in turn, believed it had a responsibility to provide FDA with the results of that review. Therefore, the report speaks to the future, suggesting that if FDA implementation of the six FDCA sections under study is to continue to be viewed as adequate by its State counterparts and critics, the agency must manage the petition process in an efficient, timely manner and commit Federal resources to food labeling enforcement. The Committee views its observations regarding both the petition process and enforcement as important outcomes of this study, together with its conclusions regarding the adequacy of FDA implementation and the status of existing State requirements.

ACKNOWLEDGMENTS

It is difficult to find an appropriate way to acknowledge the many persons who contributed to the development and completion of this report. Data on existing labeling statutes and related regulations were received from the 50 States, and one local jurisdiction. The Committee also drew heavily on FDA and others knowledgeable in the field of food labeling. It is not unreasonable to conclude that literally hundreds of people were somehow involved in the effort. The gratitude of the Committee extends well beyond those few who receive special recognition in the following paragraphs.

First, the Committee thanks those individuals who made presentations at its public meeting on behalf of State, national, and public interest organizations, and food companies: Richard Frank, Sherwin Gardner, Dennis Johnson, Sharon Lindan, Allen Matthys, Dan Sowards, Merrill Thompson, and Francis Williams (see also Appendix B). Their presentations provided a solid base of information for the Committee's work. Second, the Committee recognizes the critical contribution of all those at the State and local levels of government who provided data. These individuals are not all known to the Committee, but their contributions are no less appreciated. Third, the Committee thanks the staff of FDA, especially those in the Division of Nutrition and the Regulations and Industry Activities Branch of the Center for Food Safety and Applied Nutrition, as well as the Division of Federal-

State Relations of the Office of Regulatory Affairs. These offices all provided materials and other assistance to help the Committee understand the agency's policies and procedures.

At several of its meetings, the Committee held panel discussions focused on specific issues. We therefore wish to thank the following individuals for their participation in discussing:

- NLEA background and Federal implications—Heinz Wilms, Director, Division of Federal-State Relations, FDA; Peter Barton Hutt, Partner, Covington and Burling; and William Schultz, Counsel, Subcommittee on Health, Committee on Health and the Environment, U.S. House of Representatives;
- perspectives of State regulators—Leroy Corbin, National Association of State Departments of Agriculture; Jim Sevchik, New York State Department of Agriculture and Markets; Dan Sowards, Association of Food and Drug Officials; and Betsy Woodward, Florida Department of Agriculture and Consumer Services;
- industry concerns—Sherwin Gardner, Grocery Manufacturers of America; and Allen Matthys, National Food Processors Association; and
- consumer views—Bruce Silverglade and Sharon Lindan, Center for Science in the Public Interest; Amy Karas, New York City Office of Consumer Affairs; and Barry Rubin, the Advocacy Institute.

Special thanks go to Richard L. Frank and Christina M. Markus of Olsson, Frank, and Weeda, P.C., and Sharon Lindan of the Center for Science in the Public Interest for their assistance in the identification of additional State and local food labeling activities, laws, and regulations relevant to the Committee's charge. The Committee also is indebted to Tom Mullen and Shirley Murphy, students at Hastings College of the Law, University of California, for performing legal data base searches to double-check the Committee's work, and Chambers Bryson, former chief of the Food and Drug Branch, California Department of Health Services, for drafting a background paper on State enforcement and the process of petitioning FDA for exemptions/exceptions from food labeling statutes.

Ten food companies and trade associations must be thanked for providing information on the economic costs/savings of uniform food laws and regulations: Borden Foods, General Mills, Grocery Manufacturers of America, Kellogg Company, Kraft General Foods, Land O'Lakes, National Food Processors Association, Pepsico-Frito Lay, Procter & Gamble, and the Quaker Oats Company.

The Committee also wishes to thank the Institute of Medicine's project staff who were critical to the completion of this report. Donna V. Porter,

Project Director; Robert O. Earl, Staff Officer; and Barbara L. Matos, Project Assistant, were thoughtful, insightful, and untiring in their support. Others within the IOM who were supportive of the project and understanding of its unique character were Catherine E. Woteki, FNB Director, and Enriqueta C. Bond, IOM Executive Director. IOM computer analyst Sabrina Montesa ensured proper manuscript and report preparation.

Finally, I wish to thank my 12 colleagues on the Committee on State Food Labeling. They were a most able team who accepted the challenge of reviewing, categorizing, and evaluating the plethora of gathered materials with the professional skills and good humor necessary to provide Congress with the study it requested and ensure the development of a thoughtful, useful report for FDA. It was a pleasure to be associated with them and serve as chairman of the Committee.

J. PAUL HILE, *Chair*
Committee on State Food Labeling

Contents

PREFACE   vii

1   SUMMARY   1

2   BACKGROUND OF THE STUDY   27
    Committee Procedures, 30

3   CONTEXTUAL FACTORS AFFECTING THE
    REGULATION OF MISBRANDED FOOD   35
    Developments Before 1900, 36
    Developments Between 1900 and 1940, 40
    Developments Between 1940 and 1970, 44
    Developments Between 1970 and 1990, 48
    Current Federal and State Roles in
      Food Regulation, 54
    Implications for FDCA Section 403, 58

4   CRITERIA FOR DETERMINING ADEQUATE
    IMPLEMENTATION OF THE FEDERAL STATUTE   63
    The Historical Approach of FDA
      in Implementing FDCA, 65
    Summary of State and Local Comments, 69
    Summary of Industry Comments, 71
    Summary of Consumer Interest Group Comments, 72
    Committee Deliberations, 73
    Developing the Committee's Criteria, 80

xiii

5   COMPARISON AND ANALYSIS OF FEDERAL AND
     STATE FOOD LABELING REQUIREMENTS   85
     Complexity of the Analysis and Coverage, 85
     Food Under the Name of Another
        Food—Section 403(b), 87
     Container Fill and Deceptive
        Packaging—Section 403(d), 90
     Placement of Required
        Information—Section 403(f), 97
     Standards of Quality and of Fill of
        Container—Section 403(h), 103
     Common or Usual Name—Section 403(i)(1), 107
     Labeling of Artificial Colorings, Flavorings,
        and Chemical Preservatives—Section 403(k), 126

6   ISSUES RAISED BY STATES, CONSUMERS,
     AND INDUSTRY   141
     Enforcement as a Dimension of Implementation, 142
     State Action Under NLEA, 144
     Cooperative Relationships Between FDA
        and the States, 147
     Preemption and the Petition Process, 149
     Economic Impact of Nonuniformity, 153
     Committee Observations, 159

APPENDIXES   163

A   Provision for the State Food Labeling Study Contained
     in the Nutrition Labeling and Education Act of 1990   165

B   Participants at the Public Meeting Held by the
     Committee on State Food Labeling, May 30, 1991   167

C   Letter of Request Sent to State and Local Regulators
     and Consumer Groups by the Committee on
     State Food Labeling   169

D   States Providing Written Response to the Six Questions
     from the Committee on State Food Labeling   173

E   Individuals from States That Provided Information
     to the Committee on State Food Labeling   175

F   State and Local Laws, Regulations, and Other
     Materials Submitted to the Committee on State
     Food Labeling   183

G   Areas of Discrepancy Between Federal and State Food
     Labeling Requirements Identified by States and
     Consumer and Industry Groups   195

H   State Food Labeling Requirements and Relationship
     to the Misbranding Provisions of Section 403 of
     the Federal Food, Drug, and Cosmetic Act   203

I   Case Study: Requirements for Labeling Bottled Water   209

J   Biographical Sketches of Committee Members and Staff   219

INDEX   225

1

Summary

On November 8, 1990, President Bush signed into law the Nutrition Labeling and Education Act (NLEA), which mandated nutrition labeling information on most foods marketed to American consumers. The Act also provided for a nationally uniform food labeling regulatory system, which was to be achieved by preempting State and local labeling requirements whose coverage overlapped with certain provisions of the Federal Food, Drug, and Cosmetic Act of 1938 (FDCA). In passing the legislation, Congress concluded that to achieve the goal of national uniform food labeling, certain State and local requirements should be preempted. Based on this consideration, all State and local requirements of the type contained in FDCA Section 403 were preempted on a schedule that varied over a 24-month period. For six provisions of FDCA Section 403, however, Congress concluded that further study was needed to determine whether those provisions had been adequately implemented by the Food and Drug Administration (FDA) and whether any State or local requirements should be considered for Federal adoption. Preemption of State and local requirements related to those six provisions of FDCA Section 403 was to occur only after a study had been conducted. This report is the culmination of that study, the purpose of which was to review and determine whether current Federal requirements were adequately implementing the intent of the six provisions of FDCA Section 403.

NLEA directed the Secretary of the U.S. Department of Health and Human Services (DHHS), through FDA, to implement such a study. FDA thus contracted with the Institute of Medicine (IOM) to study the adequacy of implementation of the following provisions: FDCA Sections 403(b) [food sold under the name of another food], 403(d) [misleading container], 403(f) [prominence of required information], 403(h) [standards of quality and fill],

403(i)(1) [common or usual name], and 403(k) [labeling of artificial flavorings, colorings, or chemical preservatives]. The IOM established the Committee on State Food Labeling under the auspices of the Food and Nutrition Board to advise the agency on whether those six provisions of the law were being adequately implemented and recommend any State requirements that should be considered for Federal adoption. The charge to the Committee was to

- assemble a listing of all relevant State and local laws and regulations dealing with six misbranding sections of FDCA specified for study in NLEA;
- describe the provisions of each of the relevant State and local statutes that pertain to the sections under study and the basis on which those provisions were developed; and
- assess the extent to which each of the six sections of FDCA is being implemented under current and proposed regulations and evaluate existing data on the impact of such implementation on public health and nutrition.

This report is the product of the Committee's research, analysis, and deliberations; the findings and conclusions presented are based on materials received from FDA, State and local food officials, industry trade associations and companies, and consumer groups; presentations to the Committee; correspondence; and searches of legal data bases. The Committee's assignment turned out to be a good deal more complex than it initially appeared and entailed the deciphering of Federal requirements, discovery and classification of State requirements, translation of Congress's somewhat delphic language about adequacy and implementation, and determined pursuit of an understanding of the purpose and impact of State requirements. The Committee developed well-defined working principles and criteria for analysis and viewed its jurisdiction rather broadly in its efforts to untangle many of these complexities.

As a consequence of the lack of clear lines separating some of the six study provisions, the Committee had to classify and review State food labeling requirements based upon the exercise of its best judgment. Based on the legislative history and text of the NLEA, the Committee excluded from its deliberations issues related to food safety, grading, kosher, organic, natural, origin, and open date labeling; which were not preempted under the Act. The Committee also excluded an analysis of emerging State and local regulatory issues such as environmental "green" labeling, although it believes these issues deserve consideration by FDA in the future.

CONTEXTUAL FACTORS AFFECTING THE
REGULATION OF MISBRANDED FOOD

From the beginning of the twentieth century, and certainly since passage of FDCA, there has been a tremendous change in the types of food products available to the American consumer. A brief review of the progress made in the past 50 years provides a sense of the significant differences that exist in today's food products and the marketplace compared with those of 1938. Indeed, the complex national and international systems for food manufacturing and merchandising have been a significant factor behind the impetus for national control of food regulation.

The evolution of food products cannot be considered separately from the significant changes that have occurred in food packaging. A related factor is the importance of package design and graphics, which in today's market are fundamental to product differentiation on the shelf. Manufacturers see "burdensome" labeling requirements as a potential obstacle to the marketability of their products—not only domestically but in international food trade, an area of substantial marketing opportunity.

Proper labeling to provide the consumer with useful, factual information was the rationale for the original FDCA misbranding provisions, and that motivation has not changed in more than half a century. Early misbranding provisions were related to "food sold under the name of another food"; they were designed to give consumers accurate information about the food they were purchasing. Current labeling concerns about nutrient content and health claims focus on the content and composition of food products as these components relate to contemporary public health issues.

Early in the twentieth century, Congress enacted the first Federal statute to deal with food regulation, the Pure Food and Drugs Act of 1906. This early law defined those products that were to be considered foods and contained provisions on the adulteration and misbranding of food products. The passage of FDCA in 1938 addressed a host of practices that were new or had not been controlled under the earlier statute. The Act described in much more specific terms the circumstances under which a food was to be considered adulterated or misbranded under the law and provided FDA with new authority to combat violations. Following enactment of FDCA, the agency developed "standards of identity" for several hundred foods and sought to implement the other provisions through various means.

In the early 1970s, following recommendations of the White House Conference on Food, Nutrition and Health, the Federal government developed the current system of nutrition labeling in the United States. Late in the decade, FDA, the U.S. Department of Agriculture, and the Federal Trade Commission reviewed existing U.S. food labeling requirements to determine whether those provisions were still appropriate. Although the agencies prepared detailed recommendations for implementing changes in many aspects of food labeling, a lack of scientific consensus and the prevailing deregulatory environment would not support comprehensive reform at that time.

Criticism of the type of information on food labels escalated in the 1980s as scientific investigations convincingly demonstrated the relationship between dietary habits and the prevalence of chronic diseases. American consumers became increasingly attentive to choices among foods and sought improved information on the products that they were selecting. In addition, the proliferation of health claims being made for foods created a demand for more consistent and scientifically sound messages on labels. By 1990, efforts to reform the current policy on food labeling, especially in regard to nutrition information, were being pursued by the Federal agencies and Congress. The food industry was particularly concerned about national uniformity in food regulation. All of these efforts culminated in the passage of NLEA.

CRITERIA FOR DETERMINING ADEQUATE IMPLEMENTATION OF THE FEDERAL STATUTE

In carrying out its charge, the Committee evaluated the adequacy of FDA's implementation of the six provisions of FDCA Section 403 by first applying principles developed during its deliberative process.

1. The definition of adequate as "equal to, proportionate to, or fully sufficient for a specified or implied requirement" was used as a foundation for decisions.
2. The intent of any section and any regulation, as interpreted by the Committee, was a consideration, including, as appropriate, a consideration of the impact of FDCA Sections 403(a)(1), 403(e), and 403(i)(2) when used in conjunction with the six provisions that were the subject of the study.
3. The absence of an FDA implementing regulation would not lead to an automatic conclusion that implementation was inadequate.
4. The level of enforcement would not be a consideration in determining adequacy of implementation.
5. The strictest requirement, whether Federal, State, or local, would not always be recommended for adoption as the national standard.

6. The Committee limited its study of the six FDCA Sections to any implementing regulations for which rulemaking had been completed and advisory opinions had been published, as defined in 21 CFR §10.85.

7. In reviewing State and local requirements and their relationship to the six provisions of FDCA Section 403 under study, the Committee viewed its own jurisdiction broadly to ensure a fair, balanced review of the materials provided by State and local officials and other interested persons.

Once the principles for evaluating adequacy were established, the Committee interpreted adequacy of implementation in the following manner. In some circumstances where only a law existed, the law alone could be judged to adequately implement the provision. In other circumstances, the existence of implementing regulations for a given section of the law could be judged to represent adequate implementation of the statute. In other situations, consideration could be given to other types of evidence to assist in judging adequate implementation of a provision of the law; i.e., an FDA advisory opinion.

Two additional concepts that could be used to define adequate implementation are compliance and enforcement. Compliance would address the extent to which manufacturers have met the provisions of laws and regulations; i.e., the degree to which food labels in the marketplace comply with Federal labeling requirements. An evaluation of enforcement would address the extent to which FDA has pursued manufacturers that market products with labels that do not meet Federal requirements. With regard to compliance as a measure of adequate implementation, this criterion was considered to be important because it represents the effectiveness of existing requirements to fulfill the Congressional mandate on the six FDCA misbranding provisions under study. However, the Committee received no information on compliance from its requests to FDA and the States. Anecdotal cases of noncompliance were cited in discussions with State officials, but no comprehensive record of noncompliance problems was available for the Committee's use. Although the Committee recognized the critical importance of compliance to an evaluation of adequate implementation, the absence of compliance data required the Committee to omit inclusion of compliance as a criteria for determining adequacy of implementation of the six provisions of FDCA Section 403 under study.

The Committee considered the question of whether FDA's enforcement of existing laws and regulations should be a criterion for evaluating the adequacy of implementation of the six provisions of FDCA Section 403. To determine the intention of Congress on whether enforcement was an issue for the Committee's consideration, it reviewed the provisions of NLEA and the Congressional debate on the issue and discussed the question with a number of individuals familiar with the course of the Act's development. No evidence was presented to the Committee that would indicate that enforcement was an anticipated criterion for determining adequacy of implementation. While the Committee believed that the issue of enforcement was important in terms of evaluating the agency's implementation record, it also recognized that FDA's enforcement record is significantly influenced by resources available and the political will at given points in time. Therefore, the Committee chose not to include enforcement as a criterion for adequate implementation. However, because enforcement was clearly a concern to States and consumer groups, and was considered to be an important issue for the future, the issue is addressed at considerable length later in the report.

Second, the Committee reviewed all of the State requirements it had assembled and evaluated them in terms of the tasks defined in the IOM's Proposed Plan of Action for the study. Third, the Committee categorized the State requirements according to the following criteria:

1. An adequate Federal requirement exists on the issue.
2. The agency has not adequately implemented the Act in the area of concern represented by the State requirement. Such a conclusion would be based on the requirement's national importance, its national prominence as indicated by the frequency of attention to the issue by the States, and/or the lack of an existing Federal regulation.
3. The State requirement meets a demonstrated local need.
4. The State requirement provides only economic protection to the industry, is without consumer benefit, and/or has no other redeeming virtue.

Beyond Federal laws and regulations, there is a tremendous variety of less formal written materials that analyze, interpret, and discuss FDA's view on its statutory mandate. These documents include preambles of proposed and final regulations, compliance policy guides, guidelines, advisory opinions, letters to the food industry, Regulatory Letters and Notice of Adverse Findings letters (now both called Warning Letters), speeches, press releases, and talk papers. The Committee concluded that although many informal mechanisms are used to implement the law, it would not be possible or appropriate to examine all such materials in determining the adequacy of implementation. However, the Committee did view advisory opinions (as defined in 21 CFR §10.85) as representing the formal position of FDA on a matter and, except in unusual situations, as obligating the agency to follow that position until it was amended or revoked. Therefore, the Committee decided to rely on the following FDA materials in evaluating the adequacy of implementation of the six provisions of FDCA Section 403 under study: preambles of proposed and final regulations, regulations, compliance policy guides, trade correspondence, guidelines, and other formally established advisory opinions.

State regulation is frequently justified on two counts: (1) State requirements provide an avenue for new and innovative regulatory approaches to labeling to be developed and tested prior to Federal adoption, and (2) in the absence of Federal leadership, States have often found it necessary to regulate to ensure that consumers are protected. Without judging the merit of these arguments, the Committee relied on the following indicators during its analysis of State and local requirements:

- the frequency with which different States regulated a matter regardless of any FDA regulation;
- the regulation by one or more States of a matter considered by the Committee to be of national importance and/or prominence;
- the regulation by a State of a matter of strictly local significance to both consumers and industry; and
- the regulation by a State of a matter resulting in the economic protection of the industry, without consumer benefit.

One definitional problem had an impact on the Committee's review of State requirements and preemption determinations. Often, regulatory areas of concern to the States could not be easily categorized as relating to (1) standards of identity that are different from Federal standards and already preempted by NLEA; (2) standards of identity in cases in which no Federal standard exists and therefore may not be preempted; or (3) common or usual names that are different from Federal standards, not yet preempted, and thus subject to the Committee's review to determine the adequacy of implementation of Federal requirements. The Committee decided that it could not distinguish in any principled way among these categories of misbranding relative to State regulations. Therefore, it decided to view its jurisdiction broadly: if it was reasonable to consider that the State regulation fell within the Committee's purview, it was treated as a matter for study.

COMPARISON AND ANALYSIS OF FEDERAL AND STATE FOOD LABELING REQUIREMENTS

The following sections briefly discuss the Committee's findings and conclusions regarding the six provisions of FDCA Section 403 mandated for study. The discussion covers current Federal legal authority and regulations, the relationship of the six provisions to other FDCA misbranding sections and related Federal laws, a review of State and available local statutes and regulations, and a summary of State, industry, and consumer perspectives. The Committee's analysis of each of the study provisions is built on this information, as well as the Committee's working principles and criteria, and other information and materials submitted by States, industry, consumer groups, and other interested parties. Virtually no information on the rationale for establishing or impact of implementing State and local requirements on public health and nutrition was provided to the Committee.

The Committee found that many State labeling laws were generally consistent with the Federal statute (i.e., 45 States utilize the Uniform State Food, Drug, and Cosmetic Bill and 21 States have autoadoption provisions to incorporate Federal regulations by reference). The instances in which there were apparent discrepancies were reviewed and recommendations were made. Table 1-1 summarizes the conclusions of the Committee's comparison and analysis of the Federal and State requirements. In general, most State requirements that differed from Federal provisions involved only a few commodities. Where State requirements were established in response to an absence of Federal regulations to ensure consumer protection, the Committee suggested actions to be taken by FDA and State requirements be exempted from preemption until FDA acts. Where State requirements regulate commodities important to a State economically but do not provide consumer protection, the Committee suggested that States petition FDA either for exemption from preemption or to establish a unifying Federal requirement. Where State requirements regulate a particular local need, the Committee suggested that the States petition FDA for exemption from preemption through the petition process. Where an adequate Federal regulation is in place, the Committee suggested that State requirements are candidates for preemption. In some cases, State requirements were either already preempted by other NLEA provisions (i.e., standards of identity), or not subject to the study (i.e., grading under USDA jurisdiction) and therefore not addressed. A more extensive discussion of the rationale for the Committee's conclusions is found in Chapter 5.

The Committee reached its conclusions through consensus in most cases. In several instances very strongly held views among members kept the Committee from reaching complete agreement. In these cases, both views are expressed in the report.

TABLE 1-1 Summary of Conclusions of the Report of the Committee on State Food Labeling

FDCA Section	Determination of Implementation	Conclusion	Suggestions to FDA
403(b) – Food Under the Name of Another Food	Adequate	• Related State requirements are candidates for preemption	• Aggressively pursue regulatory options for naming non-standardized foods • Consolidate FDCA Section 403(b) with 403(i)(1)
403(d) – Container Fill and Deceptive Packaging	Not adequate	• Exempt related requirements from preemption until adequate FDA policy in place	• Consider using FPLA definition of nonfunctional slack fill for Federal requirements
403(f) – Placement of Required Information	Adequate	• Related State requirements are candidates for preemption	
403(h) – Standards of Quality and Fill	Adequate	• Related State requirements are candidates for preemption	
403(i)(1) – Common or Usual Name	Adequate	• Related State requirements are candidates for preemption For commodities and food categories examined: *Bottled water* • Exempt State requirements until adequate FDA policy is in place *Cider, cider vinegar, and other vinegar products* • Related State requirements are candidates for preemption	 • Establish common or usual name or standards of identity for names (sources) of bottled water • Consider AFDO model bottled water bill

Continued on next page

TABLE 1-1 *Continued*

FDCA Section	Determination of Implementation	Conclusion	Suggestions to FDA
403(i)(1) – Continued		*Citrus* • Preempted under other NLEA provision not part of this study	• States should petition FDA to amend citrus standards of identity
		Honey • Exempt State requirements until FDA considers need for Federal requirement	
		Milk, milk products, and other dairy products • Preempted under other NLEA provision not part of this study	
		Seafood • Continue use of *Fish List* advisory opinion as Federal policy • Consider origin definitions for catfish and other aquaculture seafood products • Preempt State surimi requirements	
		Maple syrup • Preempted under other NLEA provision not part of this study	
		Olive and vegetable oils • Related State requirements are candidates for preemption	
		Oriental noodles • Related State requirements are candidates for preemption	

FDCA Section	Determination of Implementation	Conclusion	Suggestions to FDA
403(i)(1) – Continued		*Pine nuts* ● States should petition FDA for exemption from preemption or creation of a Federal requirement	
		Poi ● Candidate for exemption from preemption	
		Vidalia onion ● States should petition FDA for exemption from preemption or creation of a Federal requirement	
		Wild rice ● Exempt State requirements until FDA considers need for Federal requirement	● Issue advisory opinion or common or usual name based on botanical names
403(k) – Artificial Colors, Adequate Flavors, and Chemical Preservatives		● Related State requirements are candidates for preemption	

NOTE: AFDO = Association of Food and Drug Officials; FDA = Food and Drug Administration; FDCA = Food, Drug, and Cosmetic Act; FPLA = Fair Packaging and Labeling Act; NLEA = Nutrition Labeling and Education Act.

FDCA Section 403(b)

FDCA Section 403(b) provides that a food is misbranded "if it is offered for sale under the name of another food." The intent of Section 403(b) is to prohibit the use of misleading names on a food when there are no common or usual names or definitions and standards of identity for the food. The Committee found considerable overlap between the provisions of FDCA Section 403(b) and FDCA Section 403(i)(1), which requires foods to be sold under established common or usual names.

The views of States, industry, and consumer groups on the adequacy of implementation of FDCA Section 403(b) all coincided, reflecting the opinion that although Federal requirements under Section 403(b) may be adequate, there is a perceived lack of FDA enforcement of this provision. However, all groups viewed Section 403(b) as virtually identical to FDCA Section 403(i)(1). The Committee's analysis did not reveal divergent State statutes related to FDCA Section 403(b).

Conclusions

Based on the lack of documented differences between Federal and State requirements, the coinciding views of States, the food industry, and consumer groups, and its analysis and criteria, the Committee concludes that FDCA Section 403(b) has been adequately implemented. The Committee further concludes that State requirements related to FDCA Section 403(b) are candidates for preemption. To promote the development and introduction of new foods, however, the Committee suggests that FDA pursue more aggressively the regulatory options that will allow the formal naming of new nonstandardized foods. Additionally, as part of its annual consideration of administrative revisions to FDCA, the Committee suggests that FDA consider consolidation of the objective of FDCA Section 403(b) with that of FDCA Section 403(i)(1).

FDCA Section 403(d)

FDCA Section 403(d) states that a food is misbranded "if its container is so made, formed, or filled as to be misleading." FDA has the authority under FDCA Section 401 to establish a specific standard for fill of container for particular food commodities and thus to prohibit by regulation any nonfunctional slack fill. The agency, however, has determined that promulgating a regulation is not a practical way to implement the congressional policy embodied in FDCA Section 403(d) for all foods (it would only be practical for those for which there are standards of identity). FDA has also decided not to use its discretionary authority to promulgate general regulations governing slack fill under Section 403(d). The agency's argument in both instances is that it is not cost-effective to establish detailed regulations governing nonfunctional slack fill for all food products or specific food product classes.

In addition to the provisions of FDCA, the Federal Fair Packaging and Labeling Act of 1966 [specifically, FPLA Section 5(c)(4)] provides FDA with rulemaking authority to define nonfunctional slack fill on a commodity-by-commodity basis. As with implementation beyond the statutory provisions of FDCA Section 403(d), to date, FDA has not chosen to promulgate regulations under FPLA.

Comments to the Committee from States suggested that they have taken the lead in establishing and enforcing requirements to combat deceptive packaging and slack filled containers. Seven states were found to have differing statutes related to deceptive packaging and slack fill. California in particular has determined that there is a need to implement additional requirements to further consumer protection in this area and adopted the language of FPLA for nonfunctional slack fill as a basis for its statute.

Comments from industry groups stated the view that, for the purposes of FDCA Section 403(d), the Federal statutory provision alone is sufficient for adequate implementation. Consumer groups, on the other hand, cited the lack of Federal regulations as evidence of inadequate implementation. They argued that Federal regulations are necessary to provide additional guidance to combat deceptive packaging and slack filled containers.

Conclusions

Notwithstanding FDA's decision to rely solely on the statutory provision of FDCA Section 403(d), only a few States have taken independent action to establish their own requirements for slack fill and deceptive packaging. In addition, a wide divergence of views exists among State officials, industry, and consumer groups regarding the adequacy of FDA's regulatory actions. States and consumer groups believe strongly that this provision of the law is not being adequately implemented, whereas industry groups conclude that implementation of this section is adequate.

The Committee recognizes that the agency's lack of success in bringing actions under FDCA Section 403(d) may have influenced its efforts in this area. (FDA has lost all court cases pertaining to slack fill.) Moreover, relatively few States have established more specific requirements related to slack fill and deceptive packaging, although some are now actively considering whether to take action on these issues.

This matter was an area of considerable debate within the Committee, and two divergent views emerged. Some members concluded that there had been no demonstration of inadequacy or consumers being disadvantaged. Others felt strongly that, within the Committee's criteria, the problems perceived by States and consumer groups alone demonstrated the existence of a problem. Ultimately, the Committee accepted the majority view on the latter position and reached the following conclusion.

Based on its analysis and criteria, the Committee concludes that FDA implementation of FDCA Section 403(d) has not been adequate and that no

single State's requirement is adequate for adoption as a Federal requirement. Given the California experience as an example, the Committee would argue that FPLA language provides FDA with a means to implement the intent of FDCA Section 403(d). Therefore, the Committee suggests that FDA consider using the FPLA definition for nonfunctional slack fill as a guide for interpreting and enforcing FDCA Section 403(d). The Committee further concludes that State requirements related to FDCA Section 403(d) be exempted from preemption until a formal FDA policy is in place.

FDCA Section 403(f)

FDCA Section 403(f) states that a food is misbranded "if any word, statement, or other information required by or under authority of this act to appear on the label or labeling is not prominently placed thereon with such conspicuousness and in such terms as to render it likely to be read and understood by the ordinary individual under customary conditions of purchase and use." FDA's regulations implementing FDCA Section 403(f) include the placement of mandatory information (e.g., product name, net weight, ingredients, name and address of manufacturer, etc.) and specifications for type size of this information.

The Committee found 34 States with statutory provisions that differed from the provision of FDCA Section 403(f). The majority of these State requirements related to the prominence of information to describe specific commodities, such as names and other qualifying statements for substitute dairy products, or production characteristics, such as "paddy-grown wild rice." State requirements frequently included specific requirements for size, style, and color of type to be used on food labels. State comments focused on differing requirements, but did not provide an assessment of adequacy of Federal implementation of the general requirements of FDCA Setion 403(f).

Industry groups commented that FDA implementation of FDCA Section 403(f) has been adequate. Consumer groups stated that although Federal requirements address many important issues related to prominence requirements, they do not go far enough to promote improved readability of label information.

Conclusions

Based on the comments received and its analysis and the application of its criteria, the Committee believes that most of the specific State regulations it reviewed are designed to protect specific food commodities or industries. Many of the products for which requirements have been established are substitutes for products of special economic importance within a State. Based on the Committee's criteria, none appeared to meet a legitimate consumer need, thereby qualifying them as candidates for exemption from preemption. **Based on its analysis and criteria, the Committee concludes that FDCA Section 403(f) is adequately implemented. The Committee further concludes that State requirements related to FDCA Section 403(f) are candidates for preemption. The Committee suggests that FDA review the results of recent studies on the readability of product information and consider whether the recommendations provided in these studies offer options to improve consumer use of product information.**

FDCA Section 403(h)

FDCA Section 403(h) provides that a food is misbranded if it purports to be or is represented as

> (1) a food for which a standard of quality has been prescribed by regulations as provided by section 401, and its quality falls below such standard, unless its label bears, in such manner and form as such regulations specify, a statement that it falls below such standard; or
> (2) a food for which a standard or standards of fill of container have been prescribed by regulations as provided by section 401, and it falls below the standard of fill of container applicable thereto, unless its label bears, in such manner and form as regulations specify, a statement that it falls below such standard.

FDCA Section 403(h) must be read in conjunction with Section 401 of FDCA. Section 401 authorizes FDA to establish by regulation reasonable definitions and standards of identity, standards of quality, and/or standards of fill of container for any food. FDCA Section 403(h) protects consumers by requiring that when foods for which standards of quality and/or fill of container have been established fail to meet those standards, they must be labeled as substandard.

The Committee's review of State labeling requirements in the area of standards of quality and fill of container raised an important question of interpretation of NLEA. The Act seems clear in regard to the preemption of State requirements for food labeling "of the type" for which Federal standards of identity exist. If the law also calls for automatic preemption of State requirements for labeling of products for which Federal standards of quality and fill of container exist, the question of whether there are State substandard labeling requirements related to FDCA Section 403(h) becomes moot. Further, it is reasonable to conclude that State substandard labeling requirements for foods that are not covered by an FDA standard of quality are not "of the type" and therefore not subject to study by the Committee. Nevertheless, the Committee decided to view its jurisdiction broadly and reviewed all State requirements regarding the labeling of products for which State standards of quality and fill of container have been established.

A number of States have regulations regarding standards of fill of container, but most do not establish labeling requirements for foods that do not meet those standards apart from the provisions of FDCA Section 403(h). Industry groups did not speak directly to the adequacy of FDA implementation of Section 403(h); instead, they emphatically stated that no State should be allowed to establish different requirements for standards of quality and fill of container. Consumer groups neither cited specific examples of discrepancies between Federal and State requirements related to Section 403(h) nor commented on the adequacy of FDA implementation.

Conclusions

Based on its analysis and criteria, the Committee concludes that FDCA Section 403(h) is adequately implemented. The Committee further concludes that State requirements related to FDCA Section 403(h) are candidates for preemption.

The Committee also suggested that because of the ambiguities of NLEA regarding preemption of State requirements for quality and fill of container "of the type" related to FDCA, FDA should consult with Congress to clarify the status of these standards and requirements for the States and industry.

FDCA Section 403(i)(1)

FDCA Section 403(i)(1) states that a food is misbranded "if it is not subject to the provisions of paragraph (g) of this section [which concerns standards of identity] unless its label bears (1) the common or usual name, if any there be." A similar requirement is found in FPLA Section 4(a)(1), which specifies that each consumer commodity—packaged food in this context—must "bear a label specifying the identity" of the product.

The Committee grappled with problems associated with differentiating between State requirements that were common or usual names, or definitions and standards of identity. Viewing its jurisdiction broadly, the Committee embraced for analysis a set of State requirements that included provisions for establishing common or usual names and many requirements related to the naming of specific foods that could be subject to either FDCA Section 403(i)(1) or Section 401 (standards of identity).

The Committee found many State requirements that differed from Federal requirements for common or usual names. The State provisions established specific requirements for food commodities (e.g., names for fish), or groups of foods (e.g., dairy products, bottled water). States are highly protective of their historical involvement in the naming of foods, either through the common or usual name mechanisms, or definitions and standards of identity. A number of States expressed concern about FDA's slow response to petitions establishing names and standards for foods and, in general, with the level of Federal enforcement of FDCA Section 403(i)(1)—which has been virtually nonexistent since the mid-1970s.

In comparison, industry groups agreed that the Federal system for establishing a common or usual name under FDCA Section 403(i)(1) is adequately implemented and all differing State requirements should be preempted. Consumer groups, on the other hand, commented that Federal implementation is sporadic and insufficient to protect consumers adequately.

Conclusions

Based on its analysis and criteria, the Committee concludes that an adequate procedure currently exists in 21 CFR Part 102 for the development and application of common or usual names for foods under FDCA Section 403(i)(1). The Committee further concludes that State requirements for the process of establishing and defining a common or usual name are candidates for preemption. However, to promote the development and introduction of new foods, the Committee suggests that FDA more aggressively pursue regulatory options that will allow the development of names for new, nonstandardized foods.

Common Names for Specific Foods

Having reached a conclusion regarding the adequacy of the Federal procedure for establishing common or usual names, the Committee discussed its responsibility to review further the States' specific food requirements. After considerable debate, the Committee concluded that because its report to FDA is advisory, it would view its responsibility broadly and review all of the materials provided by the States.

The Committee selected food categories for review on the basis of their economic or public health importance, prominence by virtue of the number of State requirements that address them, regional significance, or fulfillment in some other fashion of the criteria established by the Committee. All of the State requirements were then reviewed based on comments received from States, industry, and consumer groups, and application of the Committee's criteria for adequacy.

Based on its review, the Committee judged whether the State requirements were (1) candidates for preemption, (2) candidates for consideration by FDA as Federal requirements, (3) candidates for exemption, (4) already preempted by NLEA, or (5) excluded from consideration under NLEA. The results of the Committee's review are summarized below.

Bottled Water

FDA's original decision not to define the various kinds of bottled waters may have been correct when it was adopted in 1973, but the market for, and the public perception of, bottled water have changed substantially since then. The proliferation of products in the marketplace and the increasingly aggressive claims made for those products have magnified the opportunity for public confusion, indicating that the existing policy is not adequate. **Therefore, the Committee suggests that FDA establish common or usual names or standards of identity for bottled water and concludes that State laws and regulations that define and/or standardize the names of the various kinds of bottled water should be considered candidates for preemption after a Federal requirement is established. The Committee suggests that the Association of Food and Drug Officials' model bill be examined as a unifying basis for Federal regulation of bottled water.**

Cider, Cider Vinegar, and Other Vinegar Products

In applying its criteria, the Committee concluded that none of the State requirements it had identified met the threshold for consideration for adoption as a Federal requirement, nor did there appear to be a compelling reason for additional Federal regulation of cider products. **Therefore, the Committee concludes that State requirements for cider products are candidates for preemption.**

Citrus

After reviewing Florida's analysis and its current requirements and the provisions of the remaining three citrus-producing States, the Committee concluded that the issues raised during this review fall outside its charge and the requirements either are already preempted (juice standards of identity) or would not be affected by preemption (grading). The Committee, however, found merit in Florida's position that its standards of identity may provide additional consumer protection (i.e., through specific production criteria beyond FDA's standard of good manufacturing practice). **Therefore, the Committee suggests that Florida and/or other citrus-producing States consider petitioning FDA to amend the Federal standards of identity for citrus products, and existing State requirements be exempt from preemption until the petition process is complete.**

Honey

That 22 States needed to specifically regulate this food suggested to the Committee the potential benefit of some Federal unifying regulatory requirement. The promulgation of a Federal standard of identity and quality under FDCA Section 401 would establish national uniformity through clear preemptive action. If appropriate, concerns over the possible microbiological contamination of honey, especially with *Botulinum* spores, might be addressed in the standard of quality established not only under the misbranding provisions but also under the adulteration provisions of FDCA. Such an initiative, however, is not viewed as a high priority among the overall activities associated with implementation of NLEA. In addition, State requirements that establish grades or define adulteration are not subjects of this study. **Therefore, the Committee suggests that FDA consider the need for a single unifying Federal requirement for honey. The Committee further suggests that State requirements for honey remain in effect until a Federal requirement is established.**

Maple Syrup

The Committee concludes that the State maple syrup requirements reviewed are either standards of identity and preempted under NLEA Section 6, or grade standards and not subject to NLEA preemption, and are not subject to study.

Milk, Milk Products, and Other Dairy Products

This category of products represented by far the largest number of State requirements. A careful review and evaluation of these requirements, however, led the Committee to the conclusion that all were standards of identity and thus regulated by FDA under FDCA Section 401. **The Committee concludes that these State dairy requirements were preempted upon the date of enactment of NLEA and are not subject to study.**

Olive and Vegetable Oils

Federal regulations concerning ingredient labeling and nomenclature of blended oils appear adequate. **Therefore, the Committee concludes that State requirements related to olive oil and oil mixtures are candidates for preemption.**

Oriental Noodles

Because of national marketing and acceptance of oriental-type noodles, **the Committee suggests that the existing FDA compliance policy guide serve as the national standard for oriental-type noodles and concludes that individual State requirements are candidates for preemption.**

Pine Nuts

The Committee concludes that although this unique State provision meets a local need, it appears to serve only the economic interest of a limited commodity industry. **Therefore, the Committee suggests that New Mexico petition FDA to exempt its pine nut provision from preemption or create a national common or usual name for pinon (pine) nuts.**

Poi

In view of the highly localized and culturally specific nature of poi, **the Committee suggests that Hawaii petition FDA to exempt its poi provision.**

Seafood

Nomenclature of seafood is an issue of both public health and economic concern. Identification of species is essential in cases of certain forms of food allergy. In addition, a well-regulated system of common or usual names is vital to prevent economic deception of consumers.

Therefore, the Committee suggests that:

- *The Fish List* should be continued as a formal FDA advisory opinion to industry.
- the designations of origin (farm, river, lake) for catfish, which provide potentially useful information to consumers, should be considered by FDA as candidate for an advisory opinion or incorporated into Federal regulations.
- because FDA policies for labeling surimi-based products appear to provide adequate regulation, State requirements are candidates for preemption.

Vidalia Onions

This State requirement appears to be predominantly protectionist in that no specific justification is provided for limiting the source to the defined producing locality. However, because of the widespread recognition of the Vidalia onion name, the Committee suggests that Georgia (or any other group or industry) consider submitting a petition to FDA to establish a common or usual name for the Vidalia onion based on measurable geographical, botanical, and/or quality criteria that justifiably differentiate it from other varieties or species of onion.

Wild Rice

The high cost of wild rice makes this product prone to consumer deception through substitution and blending, regardless of its relative market position as compared with other rice products. Therefore, the Committee suggests that FDA issue a formal advisory opinion or establish a common or usual name regulation defining wild rice in terms of its botanical name(s). Current State requirements should not be candidates for exemption from preemption until a formal FDA requirement is in place.

FDCA Section 403(k)

FDCA Section 403(k) provides that a food is misbranded

if it bears or contains any artificial flavoring, artificial coloring, or chemical preservative, unless it bears labeling stating that fact: *Provided,* That to the extent that compliance with the requirements of this paragraph is impracticable, exemptions shall be established by regulation promulgated by the Secretary. The provisions of this paragraph and paragraphs (g) and (i) with respect to artificial coloring shall not apply in the case of butter, cheese, or ice cream. The provisions of this paragraph with respect to chemical preservatives shall not apply to a pesticide chemical when used in or on a raw agricultural commodity which is the produce of the soil.

States have many specific requirements related to artificial colors, flavors, and chemical preservatives. However, many State provisions relate to the safety of these food additives and/or prescribe health-related warnings on food labels, apart from general label disclosure requirements. These types of requirements are exempt from NLEA preemption provisions.

More than one-third of the States reported requirements identical to FDA requirements for food additive labeling related to FDCA Section 403(k). Half of the States reported differences between some specific Federal and State requirements in this area. In addition, FDA is currently in the process of promulgating requirements regarding label disclosures for certified color additives, as part of NLEA. Nonetheless, States made few comments on the adequacy of FDA implementation of Section 403(k).

Industry groups concurred that FDCA requirements under Section 403(k) are adequately implemented, noting that a lack of perceived problems over the years provides the rationale for preemption of State requirements for food labeling "of the type" provided by this provision. Consumer groups, however, stated that Federal implementation has been inadequate, citing State requirements as offering a significantly higher level of consumer protection than that afforded by FDA requirements. They did not comment directly on the adequacy of the requirements themselves except in instances in which safety issues were involved.

Conclusions

For many State labeling requirements for food additives, colors, and chemical preservatives, there are not clear delineations among economic adulteration, health and safety issues, and misbranding requirements. It is clear however, that State requirements that specifically address issues of adulteration, in contrast to misbranding, are not preempted under NLEA. Many issues addressed by specific State requirements will either be covered by the proposed implementing rules or not be subject to preemption under NLEA.

Based on its analysis, criteria, and current FDA regulatory activity, the Committee concludes that FDCA Section 403(k) is adequately implemented. The Committee further concludes that State requirements related to FDCA Section 403(k) are candidates for preemption.

ISSUES RAISED BY STATES, CONSUMERS, AND INDUSTRY

In the process of obtaining information from States, localities, food and drug officials, industry, and consumer groups, the Committee received comments on a number of issues that were not directly related to its specific charge. The Committee felt, however, that these issues were germane to uniform food labeling regulation and devoted considerable discussion to their significance in relation to the central topics of the study.

When the groups named above were asked if there were issues other than the six provisions under study that the Committee should consider as it deliberated on recommendations for preemption of State/local requirements, the following concerns were raised:

- The adequacy of the fiscal and personnel resources applied by FDA in enforcing its food labeling requirements as a dimension of implementation.
- The importance of the enforcement activities of the States to ensure consumer protection in the area of food labeling.
- The value of existing cooperative relationships between FDA and the States, which have been developed and strengthened over many years.
- The concerns of States about FDA's implementation of the petition process of NLEA for exemption of a State requirement from preemption and State enforcement of Federal requirements, so that these processes will be uncomplicated and well managed.
- The economic cost of nonuniformity and the potential savings to be realized through increased national uniform food labeling (a particular concern of the food industry).

State officials and consumer groups commented on the importance of enforcement and the States' future role in food labeling regulation under the provisions of NLEA. Concern focused on the need for an equal partnership between States and FDA to implement and enforce Federal food labeling laws and regulations. Virtually all such comments by these groups linked adequacy of implementation with enforcement and the availability of fiscal resources and shared the concern that without a clear and important State role, many legislatures might cease to fund food regulatory programs at the State and local levels.

State officials also raised the issue of their continued role in enforcement of the Federal statute, which allows them to bring civil enforcement proceedings within their jurisdictions. FDA's proposed regulations on State enforcement under NLEA outlined the procedures that States should follow in taking enforcement action beginning in November 1992. The Committee believes that FDA will need to follow implementation of these requirements closely to allow the States to play an effective role in enforcement. It also seems reasonable that some mechanism should be established for States to apprise FDA and other State agencies of actions taken in State courts in the interest of the goals of national uniformity.

Cooperative working relationships between FDA and the States need to be further enhanced or expanded to address emerging issues on a regular basis. Active dialogue was viewed by States as necessary to handle such issues before they are either addressed (1) by one jurisdiction or (2) through the petition process, and would allow for early input from State regulators in the development of Federal responses. State officials and consumer groups generally agreed that Federal preemption of State requirements under NLEA is unlikely to be accompanied or followed by major new FDA funding to increase its regulatory efforts to make up for a perceived decrease in State regulatory efforts for preempted requirements. It is not yet possible to predict whether there will be a loss of State resources, participation, and involvement in food regulation as a result of preemption.

On November 27, 1991, FDA published a proposed regulation for the petition process concerned with exemption from preemption of State requirements. The petition process will serve as a mechanism by which States can request FDA to exempt a specific State provision from preemption. The proposed regulation outlined specific criteria for exemption and the information that must be submitted to the agency, which then has 90 days to respond on the merits of the petition. Although exemptions would only be granted to the petitioner State, the Committee believes that if an issue is national in scope, the agency should consider amending the Federal requirement.

The petition process affords the States a mechanism to deal with their particular needs and the opportunity to suggest to FDA those instances in which some informational requirements may be considered candidates for Federal adoption. The Committee believes that the petition process must take into account genuine local concerns basing judgments on evidence to justify exemption of State requirements from preemption. The Committee further believes that FDA must ensure that its requirements for information supporting petitions be clear to the States and the agency must adhere to its own time schedule for action on petitions. FDA can use the petition process as a way to evaluate its own activities in regard to adequate implementation of the various misbranding sections of FDCA.

Finally, significant concern about the economic impact of nonuniformity was voiced by industry representatives. The Committee requested information from a number of food companies and trade associations on the costs to industry of monitoring individual State legislative and regulatory activities; product negotiations with individual States having unique requirements; legal confrontations over individual State requirements; and retrieval, relabeling, and scrapping of products and labels. The Committee was advised that industry considered the economic impact of nonuniformity between State and Federal requirements for food labeling to be significant, although the cost figures it provided were principally anecdotal. While many manufacturers indicated that they viewed the economic impact of nonuniformity as part of the cost of food manufacturing in the United States, these costs are passed on regardless of consumer benefits. No information was available to the Committee to evaluate the costs and benefits of nonuniform label requirements in relation to consumers.

* * * * * * *

This study on the adequacy of FDA implementation of six provisions of FDCA Section 403 was undertaken as a result of the requirement mandated by NLEA. The Committee overcame the ambiguities of NLEA and established a set of criteria that it believed were reasonable for judging the adequacy of Federal implementation of FDCA requirements and making recommendations to FDA regarding the future of related State requirements slated for preemption. The associated issues of the States' role in future food labeling regulation, enforcement, and petitions were also discussed, and the Committee has provided its position on these issues in the report for the agency. The Committee believes that its conclusions, recommendations, and suggestions meet the expectations of both Congress and FDA. It further believes that the report will be a valuable, useful document to form the basis for FDA's development of the required *Federal Register* notices to complete implementation of the NLEA provisions for national uniform nutrition labeling.

2

Background of the Study

Food labeling is a sharing of information between the food industry and consumers. One of the most important underlying rationales for this transfer of information is the assumption that it aids consumers in making dietary decisions conducive to health. The importance of this decisionmaking has been brought into stark relief in the past two decades by changes in the desire to protect and enhance the health of Americans. Among the most prominent of these changes is greater recognition of personal responsibility, which requires responsible and enlightened decisions by each individual, as a key to good health. Evidence of this perspective abounds in the growing interest in good nutrition practices and related health promotion behaviors.

Efforts to protect health and provide accurate information about foods being purchased led to the early local and subsequent State food laws in the United States. With technological advances and increased mobility of food products, Federal laws were enacted to protect consumers nationwide. First, the Pure Food and Drugs Act of 1906 (PFDA; P.L. 59-384) and then the Federal Food, Drug, and Cosmetic Act of 1938 (FDCA; P.L. 75-717) provided the Food and Drug Administration (FDA) with the authority to regulate the information that appeared on food containers. Regulations promulgated under the provisions of these two statutes were designed to ensure that consumers received accurate information about the foods that they purchased. By 1990, however, the law and implementing regulations for the labeling of foods that had been created to address problems earlier in the century were out of date for assisting consumers to make informed dietary choices that would affect their health.

As a result, legislation was enacted to overhaul food labeling in general and nutrition labeling in particular. During the Congressional debate, food manufacturers voiced particular concern about the complex array of State

27

and local food laws and regulations that required their compliance. Industry maintained that national uniformity of both food safety and labeling requirements was a necessary component of reform to gain their support for passage of new labeling legislation. In the end, the legislation provided for national uniformity of food labeling, with an exemption for State food safety requirements.

On November 8, 1990, President Bush signed the Nutrition Labeling and Education Act (NLEA). The new law was concerned specifically with FDA's food labeling authority, addressing issues similar to those already under review by the agency. The law required mandatory nutrition labeling on most packaged foods and voluntary nutrition information for produce and seafood; specified the nutrient content information that must appear on the label; provided for certain descriptive terms to be defined and claims to be allowed; established a petition mechanism for additional nutrient and health-related claims; required that consumer education be undertaken; provided for State enforcement of Federal requirements where the Federal government has not acted; revised certain requirements for ingredient listings and standards of identity; and specified the effective dates for implementation of various provisions of the Act.

In addition, and of central significance to this study, enactment of NLEA established for the first time specific statutory provisions for achieving national uniformity of labeling requirements for foods subject to the provisions of FDCA. The purpose of Congress in this action is reflected in the title of NLEA Section 6, "national uniform nutrition labeling." The Act preempted State and local statutes and regulations whose coverage overlapped with and were different from certain FDCA provisions. State or local requirements identical to FDCA provisions are not preempted. Implementation dates for preemption varied. Some State and local misbranding statutes (e.g., standards of identity, imitation labeling) were preempted upon passage of the Act; a second group of statutes (e.g., net weight, ingredient labeling) were to be preempted in 12 months. For a third category, which included requirements for labeling "of the type" required by six provisions of FDCA Section 403, the Act delayed preemption of State and local requirements and mandated FDA to undertake a study to determine whether there was adequate implementation of the Federal law (Appendix A). The provisions to be studied included Sections 403(b) [food sold under the name of another food], 403(d) [misleading container], 403(f) [prominence of required information], 403(h) [standards of quality and fill], 403(i)(1) [common or usual name], and 403(k) [labeling of artificial flavorings, colorings, or chemical preservatives]. A fourth group of statutes (e.g., nutrition labeling, label claims) was to be preempted on completion of FDA's rulemaking process.

The following list summarizes the schedule of preemption provisions under NLEA.

- Preemption on date of enactment (November 8, 1990)
  - Standards of identity [Section 403(g)]
  - Imitation foods [Section 403(c)]
- Preemption within 12 months of enactment (November 8, 1991)
  - Manufacturer's name and address [Section 403(e)(1)]
  - Net weight [Section 403(e)(2)]
  - Ingredient labeling [Section 403(i)(2)]
- Preemption once mandated study is completed (November 8, 1992)
  - Food sold under the name of another food [Section 403(b)]
  - Misleading container [Section 403(d)]
  - Prominence of required label information [Section 403(f)]
  - Standards of quality and fill [Section 403(h)]
  - Common or usual name [Section 403(i)(1)]
  - Labeling of artificial flavorings, colorings, or chemical preservatives [Section 403(k)]
- Preemption once FDA has promulgated new regulations (May 8, 1993)
  - Nutrition labeling [Section 403(q)]
  - Nutrient content and health claims [Section 403(r)]

NLEA also allowed States to petition for exemption from preemption of its food laws and regulations. When a State or locality submits a petition to the agency, the Secretary may exempt from preemption any State or local requirement that meets the following conditions:

1. it would not cause any food to be in violation of any applicable requirement under Federal law;
2. it would not unduly burden interstate commerce; and
3. it is designed to address a particular need for information that is not met by the requirements of the sections that are otherwise preempted.

States were also given authority to bring civil enforcement proceedings under certain provisions of FDCA Section 403 with prior notification to FDA, as long as the agency is not actively involved in or has not completed such an enforcement action.

In accordance with the NLEA provisions, FDA contracted with the Institute of Medicine to conduct the mandated study of the six provisions of FDCA Section 403 in the third preemption category noted above. The study was to determine whether the Federal law was adequately implemented and examine those State and local laws and regulations slated for preemption in comparison to the Federal requirements. Based on the above review, the Committee's final report was to make recommendations to FDA on the six provisions of FDCA Section 403 under study that it determined were not adequately implemented by current or proposed regulations, and State or local regulations that should be considered for Federal adoption.

COMMITTEE PROCEDURES

Specifically, the Committee on State Food Labeling was charged to

- assemble a listing of all relevant State and local laws and regulations dealing with six misbranding sections of FDCA specified for study in NLEA;
- describe the provisions of each of the relevant State and local statutes that pertain to the sections under study and the basis on which those provisions were developed; and
- assess the extent to which each of the six sections of FDCA is being implemented under current and proposed regulations and evaluate existing data on the impact of such implementation on public health and nutrition.

To meet its charge, the Committee held a public meeting on May 30, 1991 (FDA, 1991). At that meeting, eight individuals representing State and local governments, the food industry, and consumer groups presented testimony regarding the adequacy of Federal implementation (Appendix B); they also provided supporting information about State/local food labeling statutes and regulations concerned with the six provisions of the FDCA Section 403 under study following the meeting. To obtain further information on the six pertinent sections beyond that supplied through the public hearing process, the Committee convened several panels which included individuals knowledgeable about the Congressional intent underlying the NLEA provision for the study and the concerns of consumers, industry, and State and local regulators about the impact of Federal preemption.

The developments that have occurred in food marketing, public health, and food regulation over the last century, but particularly since passage of FDCA, have been significant in terms of the changes currently sought in Federal regulatory policy. The contextual factors that have influenced this study are reviewed in Chapter 3.

As further indication of whether Federal implementation of the six provisions of FDCA Section 403 has been adequate, the Committee requested that FDA provide all relevant materials about the issues under study. The Committee's process for evaluating FDA materials required a determination about which types of available documents were pertinent to the question of adequate implementation. The Committee recognized that it would need to develop a set of criteria to evaluate the adequacy of Federal implementation and make recommendations concerning the status of State requirements. The process by which the Committee established its criteria and the steps taken in choosing which FDA materials to use are reviewed in Chapter 4.

It was also necessary to review State activity in the areas under study to determine the full impact of preemption on State and local requirements, and the Committee soon discovered that there is no easy way to identify such activities. On several occasions, the Committee used electronic mail, letters, and fliers to request information from the States and selected local jurisdictions about those of their statutes and regulations that parallel the six provisions of FDCA Section 403 under study (Appendix E). At the request of the Committee, FDA twice sent communications through its electronic mail bulletin board, NRSTEN (National, Regional, and State Telecommunication Network), to elicit this information. The NRSTEN system reaches a wide audience of food and drug regulators and professional associations (Table 2-1). From an initial and follow-up request, all 50 States responded by providing the Committee with their basic food laws and regulations related to the misbranding provisions under study (Appendix F).

The Committee also sent a letter containing a set of six questions (Appendix C) to all State governors and principal food regulatory officials, selected local jurisdictions, approximately 25 consumer groups, and several national associations of food regulatory officials/professionals. The letter requested information concerning the views of the addressee on the adequacy of Federal implementation in the areas under study and conflicting State or local requirements that might be preempted. Members of the Committee also made presentations about the study and distributed a flier (containing information identical to that in the letters) at the annual meetings of the Association of Food and Drug Officials (AFDO; approximately 250 contacts); the National Association of Consumer Affairs Administrators (NACAA; approximately 200 contacts); the National Association of State Departments of Agriculture (NASDA; 30 contacts); and the National Conference of Weights and Measures (NCWM; 300 contacts). The Committee received responses from 37 of 50 States providing additional information for its deliberations (Appendix D). The response from those other than State officials was very limited. The complete list of individuals who provided information to the Committee is contained in Appendix E. Virtually no information on the impact of implementation of State and local requirements on public health and nutrition was provided to the Committee.

The Committee used legal data bases to search for State laws and regulations, primarily to cross-check information received from the States (Appendix F). It also searched legal data bases to find case law interpreting the Federal provisions under study and their State equivalents. These searches yielded only a small number of reported decisions involving Federal or State provisions in these areas (Chapter 5).

The Committee thus depended on the voluntary assistance of States, consumer and industry groups in isolating those areas in which they believed the States had been taking regulatory action, or maintaining regulatory standards, that were different from Federal requirements and consequently subject to preemption after NLEA (Appendixes G and H). Most States did not identify any specific regulatory requirements related to the six provisions of FDCA Section 403 that they feared might be lost under NLEA preemption. Some States and consumer groups, however, expressed considerable concern about State enforcement authority and the petition process, issues that the Committee has considered (Chapter 6).

TABLE 2-1 Central Contacts of the FDA NRSTEN (National, Regional, and State Telecommunications Network) System

State Officials
  Attorneys General
  Directors of Agriculture
  Food Officials
  Health Officers
  State Co-op Program Managers (information only)

Local Officials
  Major Metropolitan Health Departments
  Poison Control Centers

Regional Federal Officials
  DHHS Regional Food and Drug Officials (information only)
  DHHS Regional Health Administrators

Professional Organizations (information only)
  Association of State and Territorial Health Officials
  Association of Food and Drug Officials
  National Association of Attorneys General
  National Association of State Directors of Agriculture

NOTE: DHHS = Department of Health and Human Services.
SOURCE: Food and Drug Administration, Division of State-Federal Relations, 1991.

Finally, the Committee sought information on the economic costs of nonuniformity. Given the lack of publicly available information, the Committee turned to informal communication with various manufacturers and trade associations. The cost information requested related to industry's monitoring of individual State legislative and regulatory activities; product negotiations with individual States having unique labeling requirements; legal confrontations over individual State requirements; and product retrieval, relabeling, and scrapping of product and labels. Although the Committee was uncomfortable with the lack of specific documentation, it felt compelled to explore this issue and present the available data at least as examples of costs. Chapter 6 also presents the Committee's findings on economic costs and provides the available information on State legislation related to misbranding that has been introduced in recent years, which serves as an additional indicator of nonuniformity.

Following completion of the study, the Committee has planned for all the materials collected from States, localities, and other interested parties to be provided to FDA. This transfer of materials will allow FDA to promulgate the required proposed Federal regulation concerning adequate implementation of the six provisions of FDCA Section 403. In addition, it will allow access by all who wish to review the materials used in preparing this report and FDA's rulemaking.

REFERENCE

FDA (Food and Drug Administration). 1991. Food Labeling; Study of the State and Local Laws Relevant to Food Labeling; Public Meeting; National Academy of Sciences. Fed. Reg. 56:21388-21389; May 8.

3

Contextual Factors Affecting the Regulation of Misbranded Food

Any consideration of reforming the intergovernmental regulatory framework governing food labeling requires a basic understanding of the historical development of food regulation in general, the evolution of food manufacturing and marketing, and the impact of major public health events in the United States since the turn of the century. The shift in the balance of legal power from States to the Federal government has had a significant effect on the way foods are regulated. In addition, understanding the background to the current regulatory environment since passage of the Federal Food, Drug, and Cosmetic Act (FDCA) helps to identify the rationale for existing statutes and regulations in various jurisdictions and the need for reform.

Changes in food manufacturing and marketing have led to the increasing nationalization of the food supply, which has been accompanied by local economic protection of specific food commodities. Efforts to protect the public's health, have also increased the complexity of food laws and regulations. These changes also may be linked to determining the appropriate level of government at which to regulate food labeling. In some cases, a level of expertise or efficiency may be required that only the Food and Drug Administration (FDA) possesses. Merchandising practices, packaging, or other features of food marketing may require national rather than regional control. The nation's system of food regulation has, in effect, resulted as a response from State and Federal regulators to changes in food manufacturing and marketing and concerns about public health and consumer protection over time.

This chapter examines the major developments surrounding food labeling and provides the background for understanding the current food labeling regulatory environment and reform efforts, and their relation to the

35

goal of uniform food labeling. It presents those developments chronological-
ly in periods; that is, up to 1900, 1900 to 1940, 1940 to 1970, and 1970 to
1990, with the recognition that developments may have occurred over a
number of years and spanned more than one time period.

DEVELOPMENTS BEFORE 1900

Food Production and Marketing

Early in the nineteenth century, the development of shelf-stable food
products in hermetically sealed containers was a major landmark in the
history of food packaging. The use of tin cans to actually seal and cook a
food began in England in the early 1800s (Sim, 1951). This convenient food
package was a major step forward in packaging, providing a year-round food
supply in three-piece sanitary containers with processing built in and
preparation requiring only reheating and/or adding water.

In the late 1800s, several innovations in packaging had developed as a
result of the industrial revolution, including the metal can for heat-processed
foods described above, the collapsible tube, the folding carton, the corrugated shipping case, and the crown closure (for hermetically sealing narrow-
neck bottles). These developments led to the introduction and commercial-
ization of the milk bottle and canned condensed milk, which together with
pasteurization had a positive impact on public health and infant mortality.
Late in the 1880s, the Uneeda Biscuit package provided a consumer-sized
quantity of crackers, undoubtedly leading to the self-serve era (Downes,
1989).

At that time, bulk dry goods, such as flour and sugar, were sold in
country and general stores. As the nation approached the twentieth century,
specialty stores developed, with consumers making separate stops at the
butcher shop, the bakery, and the produce stand—that is, if horse-and-wagon
peddlers did not provide the items needed at the consumer's doorstep. The
small retail food specialty store was run independently by the owner, and
most items came in bulk form (FMI, 1986).

The Great Atlantic and Pacific Tea Company, better known as A&P, is
generally credited with creating the first chain grocery stores—the forerunner
of the modern supermarket (Walsh, 1986). Established during the mid-1800s,
early A&P stores resembled a typical specialty store: one person ran the
whole operation, standing behind the counter and handing customers their
orders from the shelves. However, in contrast to specialty stores, these chain
operations had a direct link with suppliers, which allowed them to charge
consumers lower prices than their competitors.

Public Health

The importance of public health measures applied to the community at large in reducing rates of illness and death cannot be overemphasized. During the nineteenth century, the isolation of illness was a significant step forward in limiting the spread of disease. In addition, expanding knowledge of bacteriology led to improvements in community cleanliness in the form of water purification and sewage disposal systems. The pasteurization of milk represented significant progress for the safety of this commodity, with related sanitary measures being instituted in the manufacturing, packing, and sale of other foods.

In the 1800s, a series of publications documented adulteration of the food supply and the resulting negative impact on both the nation's economy and public health. In 1850, a landmark public health report by Shattuck documented the decrease in average life expectancy at birth in America's large urban centers and identified the adulteration of food and drugs as a matter of public health concern. The report recommended that local boards of health be established to "endeavor to prevent the sale and use of unwholesome, spurious, and adulterated articles, dangerous to the public health, designed for food, drink, or medicine" (Shattuck, 1850). Following that report, boards of health were established by cities, counties, and States throughout the country. State Departments of Agriculture were also established with authority to regulate the manufacture of food products. In 1888, Congress enacted the first broad food and drug legislation for the District of Columbia, which was subsequently strengthened in 1893 (Hutt and Brown, 1985).

Food Regulation

Following the American Revolution, the nation was governed first under the Articles of Confederation, which permitted the States to regulate activities within their borders. However, the Articles ultimately failed to ensure a cohesive union because each State retained its own sovereign powers, leaving the national government without the authority to govern or resolve either domestic or foreign problems (Taylor, 1983).

A compromise made during the Constitutional Convention of 1789 allowed the States to retain their traditional powers, including the "police powers" under which they could act to protect the health and welfare of the public. At the same time, the Convention agreed that laws enacted by the Federal government under its enumerated powers would be supreme, including the laws regulating "commerce . . . among the several States"

(Article I, Section 8, 119). The doctrine of Federal preemption originated with the supremacy clause of the Constitution, under which the laws of the Federal government "shall be the supreme law of the land," giving them priority over any State or local law (Article VI, 195). Under this clause, conflicts between Federal laws and State requirements (i.e., statutes and regulations) are settled by making the Federal law preemptive of those of the States. This power applies both to State provisions that are in direct conflict with Federal laws and those State laws that interfere with Congressional objectives. Under the commerce clause, the courts have also struck down inconsistent State laws for placing an unreasonable burden on interstate commerce.

To those who opposed a strong central government and feared the demise of State governments at the time of the Constitutional Convention, James Madison argued that, for a number of practical reasons, including proximity to the people, State governments would not only survive but would remain a vital component of the Federal system. Madison further argued that the real issue was not the inherent correctness of granting power to a particular level of government but how best to carry out the will of the people. The purpose of government at both the Federal and State levels was to do the people's bidding, and when the majority of the populace spoke through the Federal legislature, the prerogatives of the State governments must be superseded (Taylor, 1983).

Actual implementation of Federal preemption has been more complicated than the founding fathers envisioned, in part because of the early recognition that certain functions of government are local in nature. The preemption doctrine constitutes a recognition that Congress allocates decisionmaking power to different levels of government, either by assuming the power for the Federal government or leaving it to the States. Frequently, Congress is unclear in this delineation, which calls for a decision to be made by the courts. Under modern interpretation of the commerce clause, Congress had plenary authority to regulate food labels. If it chose, it could oust all State regulation of any label on any food. Ordinarily, it has not chosen this option, leaving States considerable freedom to regulate foods sold within their borders, including foods shipped out of State, so long as their requirements do not unreasonably burden interstate commerce. (The Nutrition Labeling and Education Act of 1990 [NLEA] is unique in that Congress has specified that it wanted to displace certain State labeling requirements and consider displacing others that are the subject of this study.)

Consequently, during the 1800s, the Federal government addressed food problems surrounding imports and exports with statutes enacted by Congress to regulate foreign commerce in food as commercial food production and markets grew. States continued to regulate local activities of the food industry, such as retail food sanitation (Hile, 1984). By the turn of the century, Harvey Wiley was conducting studies on adulteration and labeling in the Division of Chemistry (forerunner of FDA) of the U.S. Department of Agriculture (USDA). However, there was no Federal statutory authority to regulate the interstate sale of adulterated or misbranded foods.

Even in those early years of food marketing, health officials, regulators, and the food industry quickly recognized the value of national uniformity in the regulation of food labeling. As early as 1879, E.R. Squibb strongly recommended the enactment of a nationwide food and drug law in an address to the Medical Society of the State of New York, suggesting that "it is self-evident that a law to be most effective in preventing the adulteration of food and medicine should be general or national in order to secure universality and uniformity of action" (Squibb, 1988).

Only 10 days later, the first comprehensive Federal legislation was introduced in Congress, but strong feelings on the matter of State and local versus Federal regulation led to protracted Congressional debate from 1879 to 1906. In 1903, the Director of the Bureau of Chemistry of the New York State Department of Health noted the need for national regulation of food labeling:

> [I]t is very certain that the widely differing statutes relating to our food supply in the different States have worked much mischief, been the cause of much confusion, and seriously embarrassed some useful industries. I think all who have studied the matter will be inclined to admit that uniformity in our food laws is much to be desired. . . (Hutt and Merrill, 1991, p. 996).

Several organizations had been formed with at least one goal being to work toward the establishment of uniformity. The original 1884 constitution of the Association of Official Agricultural Chemists (which subsequently became the Association of Official Analytical Chemists) stated that the objectives of the organization were "to secure, as far as possible, uniformity in legislation . . . and uniformity and accuracy in the methods and results" of analysis (Helrich, 1984). In 1897, representatives from 10 States met "for the purpose of forming a national Association . . . with the end in view of producing, as nearly as conditions and laws would permit, uniformity of action in the enforcement of such food and drug laws" (Reindollar, 1951). The Constitution adopted by the resulting organization, the Association of Food and Drug Officials (AFDO), stated that the group's purpose was "to promote and foster such legislation as would tend to protect public health and prevent deception . . . also to promote uniformity in legislation and rulings . . . " (Jones, 1912). Since its inception, the AFDO slogan has been "uniformity through cooperation and communication," but the organization's goal has been uniformity without preemption (Burditt, 1990). This view reflects a desire to use the same legal requirements while maintaining authority to enforce local laws. (Preemption results in uniformity, because there is only the Federal rule, but in that case there is also only Federal enforcement. The innovation of NLEA is that Congress provided for State enforcement of the Federal rules.)

DEVELOPMENTS BETWEEN 1900 AND 1940

Food Production and Marketing

Prior to the passage of FDCA, Americans generally preserved their own food through the traditional methods of cheesemaking, breadmaking, brewing, fermenting, pickling, salting, drying, and canning. There was little needed in the way of packaging and labeling of foods produced by these methods. At that time marketers of food had little to use beyond graphics to differentiate their products. By the 1930s food products were being marketed in branded packaging, including Armour meat products and A&P coffee in bags (Walsh, 1986). In the same period, a number of new grocery items appeared, including bread sliced and wrapped prior to sale and frozen foods (Lund, 1989). Air conditioning of factories allowed dried products to be prepared, packaged, and distributed, leading to the development of such products as gelatin desserts, which were marketed for the first time.

Up through the 1930s, the primary materials used for packaging were paper, paperboard, or tinplate, although glass was beginning to be an important packaging material. Early in the century, the use of corrugated paper containers to replace the wooden box became widespread (Downes, 1989). (Today, paper, paperboard, and corrugated paper are the leading U.S. packaging materials.)

The designation of first self-serve grocery store has been attributed to Piggly-Wiggly, which opened in Memphis, Tennessee, in 1916 (Consumer Reports, 1986). This store was laid out with four aisles for shoppers to walk through to view and select from its 600 items. By the 1920s, the trend toward combination stores had begun, and grocers began stocking meats and perishables because shoppers preferred to make all their food purchases at a single location. By 1930, the national and regional chains were small stores, selling meats; canned goods; dairy products; bulk and packaged cookies, crackers, and bread; and a limited assortment of produce in season (FMI, 1986).

Public Health

At the beginning of the twentieth century, life expectancy was 49 years. It had increased to about 60 years by the 1930s and to more than 70 years by the 1960s. In 1990, life expectancy reached about 75 years (DHHS/PHS/CDC/NCHS, 1991). These changes were due in part to improvements in sanitation, control of infectious disease, and knowledge of nutrition (Meredith, 1932). It became more widely recognized that the food Americans were eating had an important effect on their health. One result of this awareness was that the Federal government took over control of the safety of the food supply by preventing the interstate transportation of unfit food. The States, for their part, continued to be responsible for food within their respective borders. During Congressional action on the legislation that subsequently became the 1906 Pure Food and Drugs Act, a witness representing a large food distributing company, who appeared before the House Committee on Interstate and Foreign Commerce to oppose passage of the pending food bill, declared that the food industry of the country rested on fraud and deception. "Make us leave preservatives and coloring matter out of our food," he declared, "and call our products by the right name and you will bankrupt every food industry in the country" (Wiley, 1914). Wiley suggested that manufacturers and dealers who would otherwise have made pure and properly branded goods were forced by unfair competition to practice the arts of adulteration and misbranding.

During the same period, work of U.S. Public Health Service scientists on the dietary cause of pellagra—a disease resulting from a deficiency of niacin—brought into sharp focus the public health importance of good nutrition and added a new responsibility to the mission of public health officials, which earlier had been limited to sanitation and adulteration. The first 40 years of this century constituted the era of discovery of the nutrition deficiency diseases and isolation of the responsible nutrients (Erdman, 1989).

A book published prior to the enactment of FDCA evaluated public health problems in terms of the debit and credit sides of the scientific ledger. It suggested that the problems that still remained on the debit side were polio, encephalitis, influenza, and cancer. On the credit side, it listed smallpox vaccination; antitoxin, toxin-antitoxin, and one-dose toxoid for diphtheria; typhoid and yellow fever vaccines; antilockjaw serum; vitamins for scurvy, rickets, and pellagra; and sanitary knowledge to keep foods and water supplies germ free (Davis, 1934). The author reported on a series of cases of "disease of bad plumbing" that occurred in Chicago in the early 1930s in which food handlers were contaminating food as a result of the use of contaminated water.

An early home health book of the period suggested that:

> The addition of any substance to an article of food may constitute a fraud on our pockets without causing us other injury, but in many cases adulteration of food and drugs is hurtful to the health. Milk, for example, may be the sole food of infants or invalids and these will run the risk of malnutrition if, as is sometimes done, some of the cream is removed and water added to bring down the specific gravity of the milk to that of milk which retains the whole cream. Milk containing preservatives must not be sold (Robinson, 1939, p. 20).

At that time, books and magazines on health frequently provided information on food adulteration and the problems that consumers should look for (Barkan, 1985). One volume on health and diet described food adulteration as being of two kinds: injurious and noninjurious. The noninjurious type of adulteration was classified as

1. conventional—to suit the taste and demands of the public, usually done by use of coloring or bleaching, which could be harmful.
2. accidental or incidental—arising from the environment, carelessness, or incompetency on the part of the manufacturer and usually consisting of an admixture of some foreign substance, such as husks, stems, or leaves.
3. intentional—for purposes of gain and competition (Friedenwald & Ruhrah, 1913, p. 222).

Food Regulation

In the early 1900s, the food industry strongly supported national food legislation in order to obtain national uniformity in regulatory requirements to build credibility for the food supply. After considerable debate on the constitutionality question surrounding States' rights, Congress enacted the Pure Food and Drugs Act of 1906. This law was the first national effort to regulate food and drugs by prohibiting the adulteration or misbranding of these products. The Act defined food as including "all articles used for food, drink, confectionery, or condiment by man or other animals, whether simple, mixed, or compound."

One of the goals of the law was to establish national uniformity to reduce confusion in the marketplace. Consistent with the food industry's support for passage of the legislation, the House report stated that

> the laws and regulations of the different States are diverse, confusing, and often contradictory. What one State now requires the adjoining State may forbid. Our food products are not raised principally in the States of their consumption.
> State boundary lines are unknown in our commerce, except by reason of local regulation and laws, such as State pure-food laws. It is desirable, as far as possible,

that the commerce between the States be unhindered. One of the hoped-for good results of a national law on the subject of pure foods is the bringing about of a uniformity of laws and regulations on the part of the States within their own several borders (U.S. Congress, 1906).

In spite of these intentions, passage of the 1906 Act did not secure national uniformity in food regulation. The Act did not establish the basis for a comprehensive national regulatory scheme because it applied only to regulation of foods in unbroken packages in interstate commerce—and then only to the actual label of the product. Once the food package was broken, and many packages continued to be in large bulk containers, the States had authority over the sale of the product. In a number of cases, the courts upheld State regulations that imposed requirements different from or in addition to those imposed by the Federal government.

By contrast, early statutes to regulate meat and poultry products dealt with the issue of uniformity. The 1907 Meat Inspection Act required post-mortem inspection of all animals and meat prepared for human consumption and transported in interstate commerce (Olsson and Johnson, 1984). The legislation also gave USDA the authority to supervise both processing and labeling of all meat products, and preempted State requirements for those products when moved in interstate commerce. Prior label approval was required for the marketing of meat products. In the mid-1920s, USDA established a voluntary poultry inspection program.

The 1921 Annual Report of the USDA Bureau of Chemistry pointed out that both officials and manufacturers complained of the lack of uniformity in the exercise of food control by Federal and State governments:

Lack of uniformity increases the costs of doing business, and the increased cost is usually passed on to the consumer. It arises not merely from differences in the various laws but also from differences in the interpretation of the laws by the officials in the application by them of different standards to the same product in different jurisdictions (USDA, 1921, p. 7).

Concerns about the problem of nonuniform food requirements have, however, persisted to the present, as indicated by an average of one speech on the subject given annually at the AFDO conference (Burditt, 1990).

During consideration of the legislation that was to become FDCA, a 1935 Senate report, in recognizing the "problem of uniformity," noted that the States had unanimously urged the Federal government to assume leadership in modernizing existing law (U.S. Congress, 1935). FDCA continued the authority of Federal officials over foods that traveled in interstate commerce. The Act defined the term *food* in Section 201(f) as "(1) articles used for food or drink for man or other animals, (2) chewing gum, and (3) articles used for components of any such article." In structure,

FDCA was a series of definitions elaborating the two basic concepts, adulteration and misbranding. Under the statute, FDA was empowered to regulate all labeling of food shipped in interstate commerce and deal with other matters relating to the safety and wholesomeness of food. FDCA also contained the enforcement remedies available to FDA. The sanctions it authorized include criminal prosecution of individuals and firms responsible for prohibited acts, injunction against such acts, and seizure of adulterated or misbranded goods; the latter sanction is the one most commonly used. FDA has also used several informal remedies such as publicity and regulatory letters, under the provisions of the Act, and recalls through negotiations with industry, which are not explicitly provided for in the Act.

DEVELOPMENTS BETWEEN 1940 AND 1970

Food Production and Marketing

With the advent of World War II came the compelling need for mass production and transportation of food to the troops. In the 1940s, mass production allowed the movement of large quantities of raw materials through production plants, and improvements in conveying led to the use of automation to facilitate production and packaging. Along with the increased need for foods for the military came the development of many substitute foods. At the same time, frozen foods were introduced on a large scale (frozen concentrated citrus juices were developed by USDA researchers in the mid-1940s), and vending machines became a new means to sell foods (IFT, 1989). Supermarkets quickly adjusted to post-World War II prosperity; each decade, store inventories grew by 2,000 to 3,000 additional items.

By the 1950s, introduction of the freestanding home freezer provided convenient storage for consumers who selected the newly developed frozen dinners and frozen, ready-to-eat bakery goods (Lund, 1989). Foreign foods became widely accepted. Increased prosperity led to targeted markets and allowed the food industry to introduce a large number of new products. One such product was instant milk powder, which led to dried milk powders, whey products, cocoa- and strawberry-milk beverages, and spray-dried coffee and tea (Goldblith, 1989). Late in the decade, the perceived need for food in bomb shelters resulted in technological advances that spurred the production of new foods with a long shelf-life.

During the 1960s, advances in equipment technology led to a high-quality freeze-dried coffee that quickly became popular (Lund, 1989). New ingredients, such as oil blends and flavoring agents, were also entering the market at this time. Foam-mat drying and related techniques improved the taste of dried milk. Enzyme technology began to be applied in food processing to develop unique products.

By the 1970s, health and organic foods were becoming regular items on the grocery shelf. This decade also saw the introduction of membrane-processing systems, which changed the characteristics of food fluids; commercial use of these systems focused on industry by-products (Lund, 1989). Extrusion of carbohydrate and protein foods was another innovation that led to a new generation of precooked, ready-to-eat cereals, snack foods, candy bar fillings, breading for fish sticks (that did not require baking), and dried vegetable and animal protein products (e.g., textured vegetable protein; Goldblith, 1989).

A major advance for the food industry came with the more widespread use of aseptic processing. Originally developed in the 1940s, it is defined as separate high-temperature, short-time sterilization (HTST) of a food product and its packaging material (or container), and the filling of the product in a sterile atmosphere (IFT, 1989). The major advantages of such processing are improved shelf life, food quality, and nutrient retention; reduced energy use in processing and distribution; reduced storage required for packaging materials; the ability to combine paper, plastic, and metal foils in packaging; and potential expansion of sales into new markets.

A more recent development introduced in the 1960s is the retort pouch, which is constructed of a combination of polyester, aluminum foil, and a heat-sealing polyolefin. Although applications of this kind of packaging in the United States, which were intended to allow thermal processing and shelf-stable distribution, have been limited to date, the pouch offers the advantages of light weight, compact size, easy disposal, convenient reheating, and energy savings in terms of processing and distribution. A significant disadvantage is the lack of a practical method for recycling such materials. More recent canning developments have included the two-piece can using draw-redraw techniques, welded cans, and lighter-weight tinplate (Goldblith, 1989).

As a packaging material, plastics were virtually unknown before the 1930s. The discovery of polyethylene and the applications developed for polyvinyl chloride during that decade marked the beginning of a revolution in food packaging. The need for and resulting shortage of all materials created by World War II led to major advances in the development of plastics and their applications. Plastic packaging offered the advantages of being lightweight, durable, and unbreakable. Added to the use attributes of plastic were the engineering advantages of mechanical performance equal to metal, ease of design, flexibility, endless moulding and functional possibilities, dispensing capabilities, barrier properties, and controlled permeation

(Downes, 1989). Although many plastics can be recycled, workable methods to sort and use recycling products are still in their infancy.

Several other advances have occurred that have affected food packaging. During the 1950s and 1960s, improved efficiencies in production, light weight packaging, and downsizing led to a decrease in the cost of packaging relative to the cost of food expenditures. Such improvements as lighterweight steel, the addition of ribs to add strength, better glass distribution, the introduction of polymers, lightweighting of papers, and improved barrier properties led to less material required per package (Downes, 1989). In addition, packaging assembly lines could operate at greater efficiencies and speeds. More recently, computer applications have improved efficiency and reduced cost by influencing design and manufacturing.

Public Health

Beginning in about 1940, the focus in nutrition research shifted to the determination of human nutritional requirements and the nutritional quality of foods. Starting with the enrichment of flour and bread, fortification of food was implemented as a public health measure to increase the intake of nutrients, and this practice had a dramatic effect on the nutritional status of Americans. In the 1960s, concerns about undernutrition in Americans living in isolated areas of the country came to national attention.

The increase in knowledge of the determinants of growth and development of children led to recognition of the importance of nutrition to maternal and child health. The fact that mortality rates from many infectious diseases such as dysentery and measles were higher in malnourished children than in those who were well nourished led to numerous studies of the interaction of nutrition and infection. Such research showed that malnutrition results in increased mortality from infection, which in turn puts an increased strain on an individual's nutritional reserve.

One of the purposes for passage of FDCA in 1938 had been to address problems associated with misbranding; nevertheless, many of those issues persisted. For example, FDA annual reports from the 1950s to the 1970s cited a number of misbranding problems that the agency continued to encounter on a regular basis (FDA, 1974). The violations reported were labeling concerns (many of which are related to the six provisions involved in this study) that continued to occur decades after passage of FDCA. Similar information on more recent cases was not readily available to determine whether these problems have continued to persist.

Food Regulation

Since 1938, the food provisions of FDCA have been amended on a number of occasions, primarily with regard to safety issues. Enforcement strategies for food safety have been built on the premarket approval concept imposed on drugs in the 1938 Act; these strategies place the burden of proof of safety on the manufacturers of new food and color additives. Statutes that modified FDCA include the Pesticides Amendment of 1954 (P.L. 83-518), the Food Additives Amendment of 1958 (P.L. 85-929), the Color Additive Amendments of 1960 (P.L. 86-618), and the Animal Drugs Amendments of 1968 (P.L. 90-399).

Prior to passage of NLEA, Congress expressly provided for preemption of State food labeling regulation under the Fair Packaging and Labeling Act of 1966 (FPLA; P.L. 89-755). FPLA required that the net weight of a food product, as well as other required information, be accurately stated in a uniform location on the label to facilitate value comparisons. FPLA specifically declared that it is the express intent of Congress to supersede any and all laws of the States or political subdivisions thereof insofar as they may now or hereafter provide for the labeling of the net quantity of contents of the package of any consumer commodity covered by FPLA which are less stringent than or require information different from the requirements of Section 4 of the Act or regulation promulgated pursuant thereto (FPLA Section 12 [1461]). This Act also authorized FDA to adopt regulations to prevent the nonfunctional slack fill of packages containing foods. To date, however, FDA has not proposed or promulgated regulations to implement FPLA provisions.

Congress amended FDCA in the Regulatory Amendments of 1948 (P.L. 80-766), expanding its jurisdiction to include any action with respect to a food that results in the article becoming adulterated or misbranded after shipment in interstate commerce. However, there was no attention to national uniformity in the 1938 Act or the 1948 amendment.

Poultry remained subject to FDA regulation until 1957. Passage of the Poultry Product Inspection Act in 1957 (P.L. 85-172) provided USDA with statutory authority for mandatory post-mortem inspection of every carcass and ante-mortem inspection of poultry in interstate commerce, with the Federal government required to pay the cost of the inspection program. The Processed Products Inspection Improvement Act of 1986 (P.L. 99-641) made a basic alteration in the law, to permit less than continuous inspection of processed products (as opposed to fresh meat and poultry); it did not, however, alter the requirement for prior label approval.

Not until 1967 was interest focused on the quality of State inspection of meat and poultry slaughter and processing plants engaged only in intrastate commerce. In that year, the Wholesome Meat Act (P.L. 90-201) and the Wholesome Poultry Products Act (P.L. 90-492) changed the rather casual relationship that had previously existed between the Federal and State levels of regulatory activities. These two laws gave USDA explicit statutory authority to preempt State regulation of meat and poultry products with regard to inspection and labeling for products in intrastate as well as interstate commerce. The States were allowed to maintain their own meat and poultry inspection programs, provided that within 2 years, each State program was certified as at least meeting Federal standards. For States that conducted their own inspection programs, the Federal government was to provide 50 percent of the funding; where no State program existed, Federal inspection would be provided at no cost to the State. As such, the legislation was a compromise to allow State Directors of Agriculture to continue to operate their States' programs and administer the Federal meat inspection programs. All of these products were to be inspected and labels were to be approved prior to marketing. This requirement applied to all products that contained 2 percent or more of meat or poultry by weight.

DEVELOPMENTS BETWEEN 1970 AND 1990

Food Production and Marketing

In the past decade, aseptic processing has been widely used in Japan and Europe, with growing pressure to adopt this technology, commonly known as refrigerated prepared foods, in the United States. The 1980s also saw increasing interest among consumers in product quality, which has led to a new generation of upscale foods, such as gourmet products and frozen entrees. Wider use of food irradiation has been approved, although it is not yet generally applied to retail products (Porter, 1989). New nonorganic-solvent techniques, including natural substances (such as water and vegetable oils) and supercritical carbon dioxide, have been developed for decaffeinating coffee and tea products. The increased use of microwave cooking in the home has led the food industry to respond by designing new products and adapting existing ones to meet the demand for products cooked or merely heated by this method. Ten percent of U.S. homes had microwave ovens in 1978 compared with 75 percent in 1989; by the year 2000, they are expected to be in 90 percent of American homes (IFT, 1989).

The major growth seen in the use of plastics in food packaging has resulted in potentially thousands of combinations of plastic components currently in the development stage, which offer a multitude of packaging options for the future. Environmental concerns, however, may have an impact on these developments, producing combinations that are more "environmentally friendly."

The most recent trend affecting food packaging and the industry has been the development of the category of freshly prepared and catered products. Systems that produce these products utilize controlled or modified atmospheres of oxygen or carbon dioxide in packaging to control microbiological growth. Thus, the shelf-life of these products in a well-controlled distribution system can be extended for a number of days or even weeks. Increasing use of products in this category, however, will require rethinking of the current national food distribution system of centralized, high-volume production facilities, because these products require controlled storage and transportation conditions. Some estimates predict that more than half of all foods consumed by the year 2000 will fall into this category (Downes, 1989).

Today the supermarket is a relatively impersonal, streamlined, one-stop entity designed to maximize efficiency and minimize consumer time for food shopping. These operations carry from 9,000 to 12,000 items in an average of 22,000 square feet of floor space (Consumer Reports, 1986). At the same time, gourmet stores are becoming more prevalent; these operations provide unique food items and more personal service, reflecting a return to the specialty store concept of yesteryear. The number of new products seeking profitable marketing niches continues to explode. Until 1981, an average of 2,500 grocery products were introduced annually. Throughout the 1980s, this number grew steadily, reaching a level of more than 13,000 new products introduced in 1990 (Friedman, 1991). With this explosion of new products, the length of time now used to judge success or failure on the shelf has been shortened. In many markets, a 3-month time frame for judging the initial success or failure of a product is common.

Perhaps one of the most interesting shifts in food distribution over the past 15 years has been in the way products are priced and promoted. As a consequence of this shift, manufacturers no longer have complete control over the geographic distribution of products; instead, control has moved from manufacturers to the product distributors and retailers. Trade promotions are conducted regionally, and local price discounts that are targeted to a specific area or company are often, but not always, accompanied by performance requirements in the form of minimum quantities to be purchased or special in-store displays. Although these local and regional price promotions are developed for good reasons, they also have unintended consequences, including the creation of an active diverting network. As distributors see large regional price differentials, they develop networks for moving products from one region to another. Distributors simply buy in excess of their local needs and move the product to their stores in another region where the discount off-list is not available, or sell to diverters who market the goods to the highest bidder (Smithwick, 1988; Buzzell et al., 1990). Although by its very nature this market is impossible to measure, estimates of its volume now range to as much as $10 billion yearly, and it is still growing (Boyle, 1987).

Once a product moves into a diverter network, it becomes impossible for the manufacturer to track, let alone control, its distribution. Products, and therefore labels, designed for one market area will almost inevitably be distributed throughout the United States. Manufacturers faced with inconsistent or conflicting local regulations therefore feel increasing pressure to satisfy several jurisdictions with the same label or design labels for the most restrictive markets. In some cases, meeting all the requirements of all the localities in which the product might find its way to market is impossible. In all cases, the added uncertainty imposes a cost on the industry and the final consumer. The costs incurred in meeting unique requirements need to be weighed in terms of the burden they create compared with the desired outcome. The recurring theme concerns which level of government should be charged with the regulation of food products to ensure that they are properly labeled and reach the market in the most expeditious manner.

Public Health

Concern about the persistence of undernutrition continued in the United States into the early 1970s, but it was accompanied by a growing awareness of the problems of excess consumption. Various public and private organizations began to make dietary recommendations on total fat, saturated fat, cholesterol, and sodium as risk factors for heart disease or cancer. By the 1980s, diet and health relationships were the focus of considerable research and debate. Although considerable knowledge has yet to be ascertained about certain dietary constituents and their relationship to chronic disease, labeling concerns have intensified as more has been learned regarding the long-term public health significance of certain nutrients.

Also in the 1980s, criticism of the information on food labels escalated, spurred by two developments (IOM, 1990). First, scientific investigations had convincingly demonstrated important linkages between dietary habits and the prevalence of chronic diseases, most notably cardiovascular disease, cancer, stroke, diabetes, and obesity. The American diet was shown to contain considerable amounts of such components as calories, fat, cholesterol, and sodium, which were associated with the incidence of certain chronic diseases. The second development was a response to the first: American consumers became increasingly attentive to choices among foods and sought improved information on the products they were selecting. Food producers and manufacturers responded to this interest by reformulating existing food products, developing new foods, and aggressively marketing those products whose composition could be promoted as reflecting the desirable relationships between nutrition and health. By the late 1980s, however, marketing practices still frequently resulted in incomplete information for making proper food choices. Health and nutrition claims, which were proliferating in the marketplace, were difficult to verify on the basis of the information provided on the existing food label, further highlighting the label's inadequacies.

A number of reports published in the 1980s reviewed the mounting consensus on the relationship between various dietary constituents and chronic disease. Most notable were the *Surgeon General's Report on Nutrition and Health* (DHHS, 1988) and the National Research Council report *Diet and Health: Implications for Reducing Chronic Disease Risk* (NRC, 1989). The scientific evidence in these two documents convinced many policymakers and health professionals that existing food labeling regulations needed to be reexamined to assess whether their provisions afforded consumers adequate information in light of the current scientific consensus on dietary constituents and their relationship to the risk of certain chronic diseases.

Food Regulation

Beyond its recommendations concerning food availability to those in need, the 1969 White House Conference on Food, Nutrition, and Health made a number of recommendations about the provision of information on food packages (WHC, 1970). Its final report recommended that FDA consider the development of a system for identifying the nutritional qualities of food. The report stated that manufacturers should be encouraged to provide truthful nutrition information about products to enable consumers to follow recommended dietary regimens. Other recommendations included the need to survey various types of consumers to determine their information needs and abilities to use labeling, and develop an educational campaign to teach consumers about how to use food and nutrition information.

In 1973, FDA promulgated regulations that established the current framework for the nutrition labeling of foods (FDA, 1973). For most packaged foods, the regulations allowed information on nutrition content to be provided voluntarily but prescribed a standard format. Nutrition labeling was made mandatory, however, on any food to which a nutrient was added or a nutrition claim was made. Subsequently, USDA issued similar guidelines through policy memoranda for nutrition labeling on meat and poultry products (USDA, 1989). By 1990, more than half of all packaged foods sold in the United States bore some type of nutrition labeling (IOM, 1990). These changes in food labels that were begun in the 1970s represented a fundamental shift in regulatory philosophy and a major advance in consumer information. From the perspective of the 1990s, however, the adequacy of nutrition information on food labels was questionable, and indeed, during this period, some consumer and professional organizations began to press their concerns regarding nutrition labeling.

Several changes were made to the labeling provisions of FDCA during the 1970s and early 1980s. The 1976 amendment to the Health Research and Health Services Act (P.L. 94-278), known as the Proxmire Amendment, was aimed at the labeling regulations for dietary supplements. In 1981, the Infant Formula Act (P.L. 96-359) authorized FDA to adopt regulations requiring that certain nutrient content, labeling, and good manufacturing practices be met in the preparation of these products.

In 1978 and 1979, several Federal agencies decided to review existing food labeling regulations in the United States to determine whether these provisions were still appropriate. FDA, USDA's Food Safety and Quality Service, and the Federal Trade Commission held public meetings on a variety of labeling issues and subsequently published a notice in the *Federal Register* that set out their tentative position on the changes that were needed (DHEW/USDA/FTC, 1979). The document addressed changes in ingredient labeling, nutrition labeling, label format, open dating, standards of identity, disease prevention claims, imitation and substitute foods, food fortification, and the procedures required for implementing the changes. However, for a number of reasons, including limited scientific consensus and a political climate favoring deregulation, no changes were made at that time. The only regulatory change actually implemented following the late-1970s reform effort concerned sodium content and sodium descriptors (FDA, 1982). Although several major legislative proposals to reform food labeling were introduced during this period, no bill was enacted by Congress.

An additional concern was the proliferation of health messages (disease prevention claims) appearing in conjunction with the sale of food, which needed more vigorous regulation than was being provided under existing policy. FDA's traditional position on health messages, which had been developed to combat health fraud, was that a food for which a health claim was made was an unapproved drug. This classification required that the product be shown to be both safe and effective for use prior to marketing. By the mid-1980s, however, food manufacturers generally had begun to use nutrient content and disease prevention claims to promote products. In instances in which claims were made without supporting data, the agency could have taken rapid action based on its view that the food was an unapproved new drug. However, the gathering evidence of the relationship between diet and long-term chronic disease led the agency to reconsider its position and announce plans to revise its policy (Hile, 1986; FDA, 1987).

Yet in the process of developing a policy to use food packages to provide nutrition information on the role of dietary changes in reducing the risk of chronic disease, FDA was faced with a conflict: the desire to provide more information but not compromise its ability to combat health fraud. The Federal government's slow pace in developing a contemporary policy on health messages because of this conflict—while such messages proliferated in the marketplace—led to the involvement of State Attorneys General in attempts to fill the regulatory gap that they perceived existed in preventing consumer fraud in product labeling and advertising claims. The State Attorneys General pursued a regulatory course parallel to FDA's traditional policy; that is, such claims required that the products be considered unapproved new drugs and removed from the marketplace (Cooper et al., 1990).

By the late 1980s, efforts to reform the current policy on food labeling, especially in regard to nutrition information, were proceeding in several arenas. Improved food label information was more universally viewed as a way to assist consumers in making food choices that would be more healthful. In the spring of 1989, major new legislation was introduced in Congress to mandate nutrition labeling for food products under FDA jurisdiction (Porter, 1991). By August, FDA, in cooperation with USDA, announced plans to reform nutrition information and other aspects of food labeling (FDA, 1989). In an Advance Notice of Proposed Rulemaking, the agency outlined a plan to elicit input from interested parties about proposed changes in the nutrition label by requesting written comments, holding public hearings across the country, and contracting for a study to address potential label changes. In the fall of 1989, the U.S. Department of Health and Human Services (DHHS) and USDA contracted with the Institute of Medicine's Food and Nutrition Board to conduct a study on various aspects of existing nutrition labeling practices.

On February 13, 1990, FDA reproposed rules for allowing health messages to appear in conjunction with the sale of foods (FDA, 1990b). The agency proposed to allow the use of six specific statements of the relationship between diet and disease and establish a mechanism by which other relationships might be approved for label use. In July 1990, FDA proposed regulations for mandatory nutrition labeling of foods under its jurisdiction as the first phase of its food labeling reform initiative (FDA, 1990a,c). These proposals also focused on reference values, nutrient content, serving size, and cholesterol labeling terminology. Subsequent proposals were to include proposed reform of ingredient labeling, standards of identity, label format, health claims, and label descriptors. By the summer of 1990, the agency also had initiated several label format studies (FDA, 1991a).

In September 1990, the Institute of Medicine's Committee on the Nutrition Components of Food Labeling released its report, *Nutrition Labeling: Issues and Directions for the 1990s*, which addressed the issues that had prompted FDA's proposed revision of its regulations, as well as other issues such as expansion of coverage of mandatory nutrition labeling to most food products regulated by FDA and USDA, presentation of label information, and legal authority for implementing label changes (IOM, 1990). The Committee explored a number of issues: the extent to which foods should be covered by nutrition labeling, specific nutrient information that should be provided on packages, presentation aspects of nutrition information, and the appropriate legal and regulatory configurations by which labeling reform might be implemented. The study did not include a consideration of the implications of changes in Federal labeling policy on State and local statutes and regulations.

On November 8, 1990, President Bush signed NLEA, which had been introduced in Congress 18 months earlier. The new law was concerned specifically with FDA's food labeling authority, addressing issues similar to those already under review by the agency. It required mandatory nutrition labeling on most packaged foods and voluntary nutrition information for produce and seafood; specified the nutrient content information that must appear on the label; provided for certain descriptive terms to be defined and claims to be allowed; established a petition mechanism for additional nutrient and health-related claims; required that consumer education be undertaken; provided for State enforcement of Federal requirements in instances in which the Federal government had not acted; revised certain requirements for ingredient listings and standards of identity; provided for national uniform nutrition labeling; and specified the effective dates for implementation of various provisions of the Act. Successful passage of the legislation required the support of industry, which had, from the beginning of the debate, favored Federal preemption of all State food safety and labeling requirements. As passed, NLEA provided for Federal preemption of State food labeling requirements and specifically exempted State food safety requirements from preemption.

CURRENT FEDERAL AND STATE ROLES IN FOOD REGULATION

Today, meat and poultry inspection programs are essentially federalized. In the past decade, as a result of technological changes, the amount of meat and poultry inspected has increased markedly while the number of staff has remained essentially the same. States that have continued to operate their own programs must annually review whether paying half the costs of running a State inspection program makes sense when the Federal government is willing to take over the program and pay all of the costs. Many States have opted for Federal inspection for budgetary reasons. In cases in which a State fails to meet Federal requirements, the Federal government assumes responsibility for the inspection of its intrastate plants. Currently, 28 States continue to operate their own meat inspection programs, and 24 still operate poultry inspection programs (Thrasher, 1991). The current USDA meat and poultry inspection budget is about $500 million, about the same as FDA's entire budget (U.S. Congress, 1991).

State and local regulatory officials have long been concerned about the lack of uniformity among food and drug laws. In response to this concern, AFDO developed and has used as its major uniformity tool the Uniform State Food, Drug, and Cosmetic Bill as a model law for all States (AFDO, 1984). Since 1938, AFDO has continued to amend the model bill to keep it current with changes made to FDCA. One major step to assist that effort was the addition of several provisions providing for automatic adoption of Federal statutes and regulations. The result has been substantial uniformity written into law by State legislatures and implemented by State enforcement officials in their regulations. If enacted by every State, the Uniform Bill is seen by AFDO as providing a sound basis for national uniformity in the regulation of food labeling. Currently, 45 States have adopted the model law; 23 States have adopted all or parts of Federal regulations by reference (FDA, 1990d).

Unfortunately, the adoption of uniform laws, codes, and some implementing regulations, and their interpretation have not resulted in uniform enforcement procedures by all State agencies with jurisdiction over food products. It often remains unclear why State regulation arises. One possible explanation may be that States see practices that FDA could address under the law but does not—or at least not to States' satisfaction. In other words, States would favor a different Federal policy. Another possibility is that States see practices that Federal requirements simply do not address or would be unlikely to address because of their local character. The extent to which State requirements can be categorized as representing distinctive, genuine local needs or reflecting different judgments on how food products ought to be labeled has a bearing on the assessment of the adequacy of Federal implementation. However, such information is not readily available. There are more than 380 State agencies that carry responsibilities similar to those of FDA, which results in understandable differences in regulatory philosophy and enforcement procedures (DHHS, 1990). Since AFDO's membership is drawn from regulatory officials in Federal, State, county, and local governments, the organization has continued to encourage and support uniformity of food laws and regulations among these various jurisdictions.

Current State activities that complement the Federal government's activities in food control are embodied in a number of programs and services. Most States have differing organizational structures, methods of program administration, and arrangements with FDA for the various food enforcement activities performed in their jurisdictions. Some States have two departments involved in these activities, but most have three. In the annual report FDA prepares on these State efforts, the food program is divided into the following 13 areas (DHHS, 1990, p. 3):

Aquatic products	Grade A milk processors
Bakeries	Grains
Candy manufacturers	Manufactured milk products
and repackers	Retail level establishments
Canneries	Shellfish
Food service	Soft drink bottlers
Food storage	Other food activities

Reports indicate that in fiscal year 1989, a total of $145.53 million was spent on all these food activities by 46 States and Puerto Rico; this figure represents 74 percent of the total $196.06 million spent for all food and drug control activities by the States. The food categories listed above are not subdivided to permit an assessment of actual food labeling activities performed by State agencies. Table 3-1 provides a review of total food expenditures by program category.

Federal and State regulators have worked together in a number of ways to promote uniform enforcement procedures. The FDA publication *State Programs and Service in Food and Drug Control* noted the following initiatives:

- joint FDA/State inspection of specific establishments or industries to effect both interstate and intrastate correction of violative practices, and for training purposes;
- FDA field office conferences with State counterpart officials to promote mutual understanding and agreement on current consumer protection priorities and planning compliance activities;
- formal training courses for State and local regulatory officials, held annually across the country in up to 50 locations, which cover food and drug issues to promote state-of-the-art knowledge and uniform inspection/analytic procedures patterned after FDA practices;

- technical and consultative assistance provided by FDA to States that have primary responsibilities in milk safety, retail food protection, and shellfish sanitation;
- development of communication networks among the cooperating State agencies and FDA headquarters/field offices;
- distribution to State officials of various FDA technical and procedural manuals and information;
- voluntary worksharing agreements under which FDA field offices and State agency managers delineate establishment and/or industry coverage to avoid duplicative or unplanned concurrent inspections;
- coordinated response plans for emergencies including agreements with cooperating State agencies to facilitate communications and decisionmaking in emergency situations related to food industries or products; and
- the State contract program, in effect for 14 years, which has had a significant impact on improved uniformity in State inspectional procedures (DHHS, 1990).

TABLE 3-1 Total Food Expenditures by Program Category

Program Category	Expenditures (millions of dollars)	Percentage of Total	Frequency[a]
Food service	31.20	28.32	38
Grade A milk	21.43	19.45	38
Retail establishments	16.10	14.61	42
Shellfish	7.50	6.81	25
Manufactured milk	6.95	6.31	32
Canneries	5.36	4.86	25
Warehouses	3.58	3.25	40
Aquatic products	3.03	2.75	29
Bakeries	2.92	2.65	40
Bottling plants	1.35	1.23	38
Candy	0.80	0.73	36
Grain	0.69	0.63	17
Miscellaneous	9.27	8.41	33
TOTAL	110.18		

NOTE: Because some States do not report their expenditures by program category, there is a discrepancy between the total food expenditures noted in Table 3-1 and the total in the text.
[a] Frequency refers to the number of States with inspectional activities in a given program category.
SOURCE: DHHS, 1990, p. 7.

The current regulations governing the labeling of food are located principally in the following sections of the Code of Federal Regulations (CFR):

21 CFR	1.20	Presence of mandatory label information
	1.21	Failure to reveal material facts
21 CFR	101.1	Principal display panel of package form food
	101.2	Information panel of package form food
	101.3	Identity labeling of food in package form
	101.4	Food; designation of ingredients
	101.5	Food; name and place of business of manufacturer, packer, or distributor
	101.15	Food; prominence of required statements
	101.18	Misbranding of food
	101.22	Food; labeling of spices, flavorings, colorings, and chemical preservatives
	101.105	Declaration of net quantity of contents when exempt
21 CFR	102	Common or usual name of nonstandardized foods
21 CFR	103.14	General statements of substandard quality and substandard fill of container

IMPLICATIONS FOR FDCA SECTION 403

Throughout most of the twentieth century, the increasing amount of food products in interstate commerce has led to persistent problems for State regulators. More recently, the increasing complexity that exists at all levels of government has expanded the areas of overlap between Federal and State activities. In some cases, the enactment of local statutes has further added to the practical difficulties of determining the actual or appropriate relationships among agencies. For decades, obsolete State provisions have not been repealed, despite enactment of the AFDO Uniform Bill. In addition, individual States have frequently modified the Uniform Bill prior to enactment or instituted their own interpretation of similar language, thus creating local exemptions to the general rule of uniformity. Finally, a number of State agencies have adopted additional regulatory requirements on an ad hoc basis to protect local interests (e.g., for indigenous agricultural products or to obtain local political support). These diverse sources of State requirements have been viewed by industry to interfere with interstate commerce and create a seeming disparity between Federal and State laws and regulations. As a result, food manufacturers that wish to market a new food product complain that they must attempt to achieve compliance with Federal requirements and then wait to see if any State challenges the product for noncompliance with its requirements.

The dramatic changes and advances over the past 50 years in the manufacturing, packaging, and marketing of foods have presented regulatory concerns for FDA and the States. For example, texturized vegetable protein products that were introduced in the 1970s mimicked tuna, chicken, pepperoni, and cheddar cheese in their appearance, taste, smell, and mouth feel. Federal regulators were justifiably concerned about the potential labeling of these products under FDCA Sections 403(b) and 403(i)(1) with the potential for nomenclature issues that these developments might represent. In response to new technologies, common or usual names were established for onion rings made from dried onions, potato chips from dried potatoes, and fish sticks or portions from minced fish (21 CFR Part 102 Subpart B).

The use of new and innovative packaging materials has increased the potential for the marketing of misleading containers under FDCA Section 403(d) and abuse of the prominence of information provisions under FDCA Section 403(f). Similarly, the use of artificial flavors and colors and chemical preservatives in the preparation of new and unique substitute foods, specialty foods, and snack foods has emphasized the importance of the Section 403(k) labeling requirements. Hutt and Merrill (1991) have pointed out that in recent years the ingredient statement has allowed consumers to identify and avoid specific ingredients, in contrast to the view in 1938 that ingredient labeling was strictly an economic issue. The very fact that the supermarket of today carries from 9,000 to 12,000 items and a new item can be introduced and withdrawn in a period as short as 3 months highlights the importance of minimizing the burden of all food labeling requirements.

For many years, Federal, State, and local food regulators have supported the goal of uniformity through means other than preemption. Although much has been accomplished, many regulators and the food industry remain concerned that the goal has not been achieved to the extent desired. For those holding this view, NLEA is seen as an opportunity to accelerate the process of achieving national uniformity in food labeling while continuing to provide for joint Federal/State initiatives and a meaningful role for States in food labeling policy development and implementation.

REFERENCES

AFDO (Association of Food and Drug Officials). 1984. Uniform State Food, Drug, and Cosmetic Bill, 1984 Revision. Laws and Regulations Committee Accepted and Endorsed. Annual Meeting, Seattle, Washington, June 19.

Barkan, I.D. 1985. Industry invites regulation: The passage of the Pure Food & Drugs Act of 1906. Amer. J. Public Health 75:18–26.

Boyle, K. 1987. Diverting product: A way of life or just a temporary glitch. Food Broker Quarterly 3:36. Summer

Burditt, G. 1990. Uniformity through cooperation and communication. Food Drug Cosmetic Law J. 45:319–325.

Buzzell, R.D., J.A. Quelch, and W.J. Salmon. 1990. The costly bargain of trade promotion. Harvard Business Review:90(2):141–149.

Consumer Reports. 1986. I'll Buy That! 50 Small Wonders and Big Deals that Revolutionized the Lives of Consumers: A 50 year Retrospective. Mt. Vernon, N.Y.: Consumers Union.

Cooper, R.M., R.L. Frank, and M.J. O'Flaherty. 1990. History of health claims. Food Drug Cosmetic Law J. 45:655–691.

Davis, W. 1934. The Advance of Science. Garden City, N.Y.: Doubleday, Doran and Company, Inc.

DHEW/USDA/FTC (U.S. Department of Health, Education, and Welfare; U.S. Department of Agriculture; and Federal Trade Commission). 1979. Advance Notice of Rulemaking. Tentative Position of Agencies. Fed. Reg. 44:75990–76020; Dec. 21.

DHHS (U.S. Department of Health and Human Services). 1988. The Surgeon General's Report on Nutrition and Health. Washington, D.C.: Government Printing Office.

DHHS (Department of Health and Human Services). 1990. State Programs and Services in Food and Drug Control. Food and Drug Administration. Washington, D.C.: Government Printing Office.

DHHS/PHS/CDC/NCHS. 1991. Vital Statistics of the United States. 1988, Vol. II sec. 6.

Downes, T.W. 1989. Food packaging in the IFT era: Five decades of unprecedented growth and change. Food Technol. 9:228–240.

Erdman, J.W. 1989. Nutrition: Past, present and future. Food Technol. 9:220–227.

FDA (Food and Drug Administration). 1973. Regulations for the Enforcement of the Federal Food, Drug, and Cosmetic Act and the Fair Packaging and Labeling Act; Nutrition Labeling. Fed. Reg. 38:2125–2132; Jan. 19.

FDA (Food and Drug Administration). 1974. Annual Reports 1950-1974 on the Administration of the Federal Food, Drug, and Cosmetic Act and Related Laws. U.S. Department of Health, Education, and Welfare. Washington, D.C.: Government Printing Office.

FDA (Food and Drug Administration). 1982. Food Labeling; Declaration of Sodium Content of Foods and Label Claims for Foods on the Basis of Sodium Content. Final Regulations. Fed. Reg. 49:15510–15535; April 18.

FDA (Food and Drug Administration). 1987. Food Labeling; Public Health Messages on Food Labels and Labeling. Fed. Reg. 52:28843–28849; Aug. 4.

FDA (Food and Drug Administration). 1989. Food Labeling; Advance Notice of Proposed Rulemaking. Fed. Reg. 54:32610–32615; Aug. 8.

FDA (Food and Drug Administration). 1990a. Food Labeling; Definition of the Terms Cholesterol Free, Low Cholesterol, and Reduced Cholesterol; Tentative Final Rule. Fed. Reg. 55:29455–29473; July 19.

FDA (Food and Drug Administration). 1990b. Food Labeling; Health Messages and Label Statements; Reproposed Rule. Fed. Reg. 55:5175–5192; Feb. 13.

FDA (Food and Drug Administration). 1990c. Food Labeling; Reference Daily Intakes and Daily Reference Values; Mandatory Status of Nutrition Labeling and Nutrient Content Revision; Serving Size; Proposed Rules. Fed. Reg. 55:29475–29533; July 10.

FDA (Food and Drug Administration). 1990d. State Law Data: 1990. Rockville, Md.: FDA.

FDA (Food and Drug Administration). 1991a. FDA Report of Consumer Research on Alternative Nutrition Label Formats; Availability. Fed. Reg. 56:23072–23083; May 20.

FMI (Food Marketing Institute). 1986. America the Bountiful: How the Supermarket Came to Main Street. In cooperation with Beatrice Companies, Inc. Washington, D.C.: FMI.

Friedenwald, J., and J. Ruhrah. 1913. Diet and Health in Disease, 4th ed. Philadelphia, Pa.: W. B. Saunders Co.

Friedman, M., ed. 1991. Gorman's New Product News. 26:1. Jan. 6. Chicago: Gorman Publishing Co.

Goldblith, S.A. 1989. 50 years of progress in food science and technology: From art based on experience to technology based on science. Food Technol. 9:88–286.

Helrich, K. 1984. The Great Collaboration: The First 100 Years of the Association of Official Analytical Chemists (AOAC). Arlington, Va.: AOAC.

Hile, J.P. 1984. Remarks before the Food and Drug Law Institute Seminar on State and Federal Roles in Food Regulations. Washington, D.C. Sept. 26.

Hile, J.P. 1986. Understanding the Food and Drug Administration's position on health claims. Food Drug Cosmetic Law J. 41:101–104.

Hutt, P.B., and S.A. Brown. 1985. Hillsborough Co. FL et al. v. Automated Medical Laboratories. Brief for Grocery Manufacturers of America, Inc. as amicus curiae in support of appellee. Before the Supreme Court. March 29.

Hutt, P.B., and R.A. Merrill. 1991. Food and Drug Law: Cases and Materials. 2nd ed. Westbury, N.Y.: Foundation Press.

IFT (Institute of Food Technologists). 1989. Top 10 food science innovations. 1939–1989. Staff report. Food Technol. 9:308.

IOM (Institute of Medicine). 1990. Nutrition Labeling: Issues and Directions for the 1990s. Report of the Committee on the Nutrition Components of Food Labeling, Food and Nutrition Board. Washington, D.C.: National Academy Press.

Jones, A. 1912. The Object of the Association (AFDO) as Defined by the New Constitution. American Food J. July 15.

Lund, D. 1989. Food processing: From art to engineering. Food Technol. 9:242–247.

NRC (National Research Council). 1989. Diet and Health: Implications for Reducing Chronic Disease Risk. Report of the Committee on Diet and Health, Food and Nutrition Board, Commission on Life Sciences. Washington, D.C.: National Academy Press.

Olsson, P.C., and D.R. Johnson. 1984. Meat and Poultry Inspection: Wholesomeness, Integrity and Productivity. pp 220-241 In Seventy-fifth Anniversary Commemorative Volume of Food and Drug Law. Washington, D.C.: Food and Drug Law Institute.

Porter, D.V. 1989. Preservation of Food by Irradiation. Congressional Research Service, Library of Congress. CRS 89-491. SPR: Washington, D.C.

Porter, D.V. 1991. Nutrition Labeling and Education Act of 1990: P.L. 101-535. Congressional Research Service, Library of Congress. CRS 91–146. SPR.: Washington, D.C.

Reindollar, B. 1951. The Association of Food and Drug Officials. Food Drug Cosmetic Law J. 6:52–54.

Robinson, V. 1939. The Modern Home Physician. New York: W.M. Wise & Co.

Shattuck, L. 1850. Report of the Sanitary Commission of Massachusetts. Boston, Ma.

Sim, M.B. 1951. Commercial Canning in New Jersey: History and Early Development. Trenton, N.J.: New Jersey Agricultural Society.

Smithwick, P.J. 1988. Diverting: Deals of Wheels. Pp. 19–20, 43–44 in Management Challenges 1988. Progressive Grocer Executive Report. January.

Squibb, E.R. 1988. The collected papers of Edward Robinson Squibb, M.D., 1819–1900. Princeton, N.J.: Squibb Corp.

U.S. Congress, House. Committee on Appropriations, Subcommittee on Agriculture. 1991. FY 1992 for Department of Agriculture. Food Safety and Inspection Service. House Rept. 102-119, 102nd Cong., 1st Sess.

U.S. Congress, House. Committee on Interstate and Foreign Commerce. 1906. Report on the Federal Food and Drugs Act. House Rept. 2118, 59th Cong., 1st Sess.

U.S. Congress, Senate. Committee on Commerce. 1935. Foods, Drugs, and Cosmetics. S.5 Senate Rept. 361, 74th Cong. 1st Sess.

Taylor, M.R. 1983. Federal preemption and food and drug regulation: The practical, modern meaning of an ancient doctrine. Food Drug Cosmetic Law J. 38:306–317.

Thrasher, E. 1991. Chief, Field Operations, Food Safety and Inspection Service, USDA, Personal Communication.

USDA (U.S. Department of Agriculture). 1921. Annual Report. Bureau of Chemistry. Government Printing Office: Washington, D.C.

USDA (U.S. Department of Agriculture). 1989. FSIS [Food Safety and Inspection Service] Standards and Labeling Policy Book. Washington, D.C.: FSIS.

Walsh, W.I. 1986. The Rise and Decline of the Great Atlantic and Pacific Tea Company. Secaucus, N.J.: Lyle Stuart, Inc.

WHC (White House Conference on Food, Nutrition, and Health). 1970. Final Report. Washington, D.C.: Government Printing Office.

Wiley, H.W. 1914. 1001 Tests of Foods, Beverages and Toilet Accessories, Good and Otherwise. New York, N.Y.: Heart's International Library Co.

4

Criteria for Determining Adequate Implementation of the Federal Statute

The Nutrition Labeling and Education Act (NLEA) established for the first time specific statutory provisions for achieving national uniformity of labeling requirements for foods subject to the provisions of the Federal Food, Drug, and Cosmetic Act (FDCA). One of the purposes of Congress in enacting this legislation is reflected in the title of NLEA Section 6, "national uniform nutrition labeling." The approach taken in NLEA to achieve this uniformity, however, is neither uniform nor specific to nutrition labeling. For example, any State labeling requirement for a food that is the subject of a standard of identity established under FDCA Section 401 and not identical to that standard was preempted on the date of enactment of NLEA. Any State labeling requirement "of the type" required by FDCA Section 403(c) [imitation labeling] is preempted a year after enactment. State labeling requirements "of the type" required by FDCA Sections 403(b), 403(d), 403(f), 403(h), 403(i)(1), or 403(k) are preempted under a third set of conditions (see also Chapter 2). For these latter sections, NLEA required:

(b) STUDY AND REGULATIONS –
(1) For the purpose of implementing Section 403(a)(3), the Secretary of Health and Human Services shall enter into a contract with a public or nonprofit private entity to conduct a study of –

(A) State and local laws which require the labeling of food that is of the type required by sections 403(b), 403(d), 403(f) 403(h), 403(i)(1), and 403(k) of the Federal Food, Drug, and Cosmetic Act, and

(B) The sections of the Federal Food, Drug, and Cosmetic Act referred to in subparagraph (A) and the regulations issued by the Secretary to enforce such sections to determine whether such sections and regulations adequately implement the purposes of such sections.

Under NLEA, the Secretary is bound by a strict timetable to disseminate the results of the study and propose changes in the Federal requirements, as appropriate. The focus of the Committee's work thus was outlined within the specific language of NLEA.

One of the Committee's tasks was to establish a definition for adequate implementation as a basis for judging current Federal requirements. The Committee began with the NLEA statutory language and examined the *Congressional Record* on the subject. This inquiry revealed that the debate in both chambers primarily centered on sections other than the provision mandating this study. However, in summarizing the requirements of NLEA for the full House, Representative Henry A. Waxman (D-Calif.) made the following statements:

> Section 6(b)(1) requires the Secretary to enter into a contract for a study of State and local laws of the type that will be preempted by Section 403(a)(3), and of the relevant federal laws and regulations. *The purpose of this study is to provide the Secretary information upon which to determine whether federal laws are adequate once the State laws are preempted* [emphasis added]. It is anticipated that the study will identify all federal regulations that are applicable as well as State laws that will be preempted. The study should also survey local laws, but it is not anticipated that every local law will need to be identified (U.S. Congress, 1990).

This language emphasized in particular that Congress expected the Committee to go beyond merely determining the existence of a Federal regulation. Rather, it was to decide, once State requirements were preempted, whether the remaining Federal statutes and regulations were adequate for the protection of the public.

The Committee also sought guidance from persons who participated directly in the development of NLEA Section 6(b). William Schultz, Counsel to the House Subcommittee on Health and the Environment, and Peter Barton Hutt, Partner in the law firm of Covington and Burling, met with the Committee on separate occasions to share their recollections of the Congressional discussions of the definition of "adequate implementation" and the Committee's charge. As a result of these discussions, the Committee learned the following regarding the development of Section 6:

- There was no attempt on the part of Congress specifically to define adequate implementation; the final determination was left to those who would conduct the study as part of their recommendations to the Secretary.
- The expectation of Congress was that the adequacy of the Food and Drug Administration's (FDA) implementation was to be determined by

the specific language of statutes, regulations, and any other formal statements of policy issued by FDA.

- Congress understood that the actual level of effort exerted at any moment in time by FDA to enforce FDCA, its regulations, or policies was subject to factors beyond the scope of the study and therefore should not be a consideration of the Committee in its deliberations (Hutt, 1991; Schultz, 1991).

THE HISTORICAL APPROACH OF FDA IN IMPLEMENTING FDCA

The Committee then focused on formal statements and policies of FDA as indicators of implementation.

FDCA and Court Enforcement Actions

FDCA Section 701(a) authorizes, but does not require, FDA to promulgate regulations for the efficient enforcement of the Act. In contrast, NLEA requires FDA to promulgate certain implementing regulations. Similarly, other recent amendments to FDCA (e.g., Safe Medical Devices Act of 1990) have directed FDA to promulgate regulations to a prescribed end on an established schedule. Historically, however, except for specific requirements such as those mentioned above, FDA has maintained that regulations are not necessary for effective enforcement of a law such as FDCA but are thought to be fairer and more efficient.

From 1938 to 1970, FDA relied primarily on case-by-case enforcement to establish principles and policies for food labeling and other requirements. From 1970 to the early 1980s, the agency emphasized regulations, particularly in the area of food labeling. This approach was typical for the period, although enforcement data reveal that such heavy reliance changed over time: FDA instituted 3,848 separate court actions in fiscal year 1945, as compared with only 843 in 1971 (Hutt, 1973). FDA continues to believe that successful civil and criminal actions establish valuable precedent for future conduct by the regulated industry. When appropriate, the agency has relied on the established body of case law in the area of food labeling, especially that created during the first two decades following passage of the 1938 Act (Hutt and Merrill, 1991). The steady decline in these types of enforcement activities beginning in the 1960s, however, reflects the increased use of the authority to promulgate regulations (Pfeifer, 1984).

The Increasing Use of Regulations

Although FDA issued some regulations prior to 1938, their legal status and enforceability were frequently challenged. The express rulemaking authority of the 1938 Act, however, began to alter industry's attitude toward and acceptance of the agency's regulations, although the substantive character of the regulations continued to be challenged from time to time (Pfeifer, 1984). Passage of the Administrative Procedure Act in 1946 established the basic framework of rulemaking for all government agencies, including FDA (Mintz and Miller, 1991). The agency, however, did not immediately turn to rulemaking as its principal means of setting implementation policy under FDCA. Thus, by the early 1970s, FDA and many other Federal agencies were subjected to criticism by the Administrative Conference of the United States for not establishing policies through rulemaking (Hamilton, 1972). In response to that criticism, agencies began to expand their use of regulations as a means of enunciating policy.

During this same period, new and innovative approaches to regulate food labeling were being proposed. Many recommendations from the final report of the White House Conference on Food, Nutrition, and Health (WHC, 1969) formed the basis for FDA's proposing new regulations on nutrient content labeling and alternative regulatory approaches for other aspects of food labeling (i.e., the common or usual name regulation instead of the establishment of standards of identity; 21 CFR Part 102; FDA, 1972; FDA, 1973).

The promulgation of rules has now become the principal means by which FDA implements its regulatory programs. During the past two decades, its regulations have become increasingly detailed in their requirements and the preambles to the regulations have become more extensive in their discussion of the agency's rationale and plans for enforcement. Regulations are now used to set standards for or otherwise define products, require specific labeling, establish procedures or define good manufacturing practices for the industry, or establish administrative processes for use by the public or the agency itself (Pfeifer, 1984). FDA's rationale in part is that by publicly establishing rules, responsible firms will comply, thus contributing to efficient enforcement of FDCA (Hutt and Merrill, 1991).

Advisory Opinions as a Means of Implementation

The process of promulgating regulations is burdensome and time-consuming. Therefore, regulations ordinarily speak to matters that are not transient or subject to frequent change. To address matters that are of importance to industry but specific to a class of product or reflective of current scientific procedure, FDA provides advisory opinions—statements of policy and interpretation of its position on such issues. FDA has formalized the procedure by regulation (21 CFR §10.85; FDA, 1979; FDA, 1981).

The first advisory opinions were issued during the early 1940s as excerpts from trade correspondence, generally known as TCs. However, after passage of the Administrative Procedure Act in 1946, such policy statements were required to be published in the *Federal Register,* and the TC system was discontinued (Levinson, c. 1952), although a number of TCs remain in effect today as advisory opinions [21 CFR §10.85(d)(2)]. The TC system was followed by a system called "Statements of Policy and Interpretation," which were published in the *Federal Register* and codified. (The remnants of this system can be found in 21 CFR Part 1, Subpart B.) In recent years, FDA increasingly has used general statements of policy in the form of advisory opinions (in response to industry requests) or guidelines developed on its own initiative to indicate its position in instances in which regulations are not appropriate. For example, FDA developed guidelines to provide guidance on conducting safety studies of new food additive products requiring premarket approval; this guidance (known as the *Red Book*) must be revised continuously to reflect contemporary scientific methods and thus is not amenable to issuance as regulations. Another example is *The Fish List,* which defines more than 100 species of fish for labeling purposes. Such guidelines provide a "safe harbor" for industry, because they are binding on FDA until revoked. They are not binding on industry; nevertheless, if followed by a company, they provide assurance that the conduct of the company is acceptable to FDA. The preambles to regulations and formal notices published by FDA in the *Federal Register* also carry advisory opinion status. The advisory opinion process is defined in 21 CFR §10.85.

Speeches, Articles, and Other Statements by FDA Employees

As part of their day-to-day activities, FDA officials frequently are asked to make speeches, write articles for publication, or informally discuss current agency activities at public meetings. Such statements are eagerly sought and provide valuable insights into emerging policies. Investigators and compliance officers also are often confronted with situations in which they must discuss their views on FDA policy.

Such advice must be accepted for what it is: an informal communication that represents the best judgment of an employee at a given point in time but that does not constitute an official FDA advisory opinion. Except in cases in which the written advice is provided and issued under the provisions of Sections 21 CFR §10.85 or §10.90, it cannot be relied upon to represent the formal position of the agency and does not bind, otherwise obligate, or commit FDA to the views expressed [21 CFR §10.85(k)].

FDA Policy on Preemption

FDA included in the preamble to its proposed rule, State Petitions Requesting Exemption from Federal Preemption, a discussion of preemption and the policies it will follow in granting exemptions. Regarding the intent of NLEA, FDA stated that:

> Moreover, section 6(c)(1) of the 1990 amendments clearly manifests Congress's intention that the 1990 amendments "shall not be construed to preempt any provision of State law, unless such provision is expressly preempted under section 403A of the Act." Section 403A of the act is only operative in matters where there is a Federal requirement applicable to the labeling addressed in the State requirement. If there is no applicable Federal requirement that has been given preemptive status by Congress, there is no competing claim of jurisdiction, and, therefore, no basis under the 1990 amendments for Federal preemption or grounds to justify the submission of a State petition for exemption. Therefore, FDA has no authority under the 1990 amendments to rule on State petitions for exemption where the 1990 amendments have not imposed such Federal requirements. Of course section 6(c)(3) of the 1990 amendments provides that the amendments shall not affect any preemption, expressed or implied, which arises under the Constitution or other provisions of Federal law or regulation.
>
> Several examples of the types of State requirements that would not be subject to the preemption provisions of the 1990 amendments were given in the Congressional Record of July 30, 1990 (H5842). The examples included State laws pertaining to issues for which there is no national framework, such as open date labeling, unit price labeling, container deposit labeling, religious dietary labeling, and previously frozen labeling (FDA, 1991, p. 60530).

The agency continued its discussion by referencing Executive Order 12612 on federalism as its guiding policy regarding preemption.

> In construing the provision for exemption from preemption, the agency is guided by the policy in Executive Order 12612 (E.O. 12612) of October 26, 1987 on federalism (52 FR 41685 at 41687, October 30, 1987) that preemption of State law shall be restricted to the minimum level necessary to achieve the objectives of the statute. A corollary of this policy is that exemption from preemption should be liberally granted to the extent that the statutory objectives are fulfilled. FDA will consider E.O. 12612 as part of its review of any petitions that it receives (FDA, 1991, p. 60530).

During its closing deliberations and final review of its draft report, the Committee concluded that it was appropriate and necessary to recognize the publication of the proposal in its report (see also Chapter 6). The Committee has not, however, gone beyond this recognition, concluding further that the publication by the agency of the proposed regulation and its preamble should not affect its recommendations to FDA.

SUMMARY OF STATE AND LOCAL COMMENTS

As part of its process of collecting State laws and regulations that might be preempted by NLEA, the Committee specifically requested guidance from States and localities in defining adequate implementation for the purposes of this study. The responses to this request took a number of different forms but can be generally summarized as follows.

The Association of Food and Drug Officials (AFDO) identified the factors that it believed influence adequacy:

> We firmly believe that a regulation becomes "adequate" only when it (1) is sufficient as an enforcement tool to prevent fraudulent or misleading claims; (2) addresses the subject to the extent necessary to provide for good, sound nutrition in all of the areas it purports to encompass; (3) uses up-to-date terminology and science to define foods and food descriptors, and at the same time meets the criteria in (1) above; and (4) omits no meaningful information which is addressed by a state or local law or regulation (AFDO, 1991).

AFDO also noted that even so-called industry protectionist requirements often provide valuable consumer protection, citing orange juice regulation by the State of Florida. AFDO believes that Florida officials have more experience than officials from other States in dealing with misbranding of fruit juices and, therefore the State requirements are beneficial both to consumers as well as industry (AFDO, 1991).

The Attorneys General of seven States (California, Iowa, Minnesota, Missouri, New York, Texas, and Wisconsin) also provided a definition of adequacy for the Committee's consideration:

> The standard for making that determination [of adequate implementation] should be whether the federal regulations in the subject areas of the study are at least as protective of the public's well-being as existing state law or regulations. Where a state's laws are more protective, we urge the Committee to conclude that the federal regulations do not adequately implement those provisions of the FDCA and that protections at least as stringent as those provided by state laws or regulations should be adopted by the FDA through rulemaking. Any other result would be to strip consumers of their current level of protection and would run contrary to the intent of the legislators who drafted the NLEA (State Attorneys General, 1991).

The Attorneys General suggested that States often serve as "laboratories of democracy," taking the lead in responding to the public's needs locally and well in advance of a Federal response. In this fashion, States ultimately stimulate the Federal government to act and provide a template for any national standard. They offered two examples of areas in which States are providing such leadership: the labeling of bottled water and the regulating of misleading containers. Special attention was drawn to the bottled water requirements of California and New York, which require labels to identify the source of the water, and the California requirement prohibiting the use of a false bottom, sidewalls, lid, or covering in a "fashion to facilitate the perpetration of deception or fraud" (State Attorneys General, 1991).

Twenty-one of the States that responded to the Committee's request reported that their State food and drug laws included an automatic adoption provision (Table 4-1). Under these circumstances, FDA regulations are automatically adopted (or adopted under simplified, streamlined procedures) as State regulations. Some States pointed out, however, that certain local problems have required special additional action by States, even with the automatic adoption provisions. In these instances, the States urged the Committee to recommend that such State requirements be candidates for adoption as Federal requirements. The example most frequently cited was, again, the regulation of bottled water labeling (see Appendix I).

Only a limited number of responses to the Committee's request were received from localities (city and county governments). The responses revealed no conflicts with Federal requirements.

TABLE 4-1 Status of State Automatic Adoption Provisions for Federal Requirements of the Food, Drug, and Cosmetic Act of 1938, as Amended

State	With Auto Adoption	Without Auto Adoption
Alabama		x
Alaska		x
Arizona	x	
Arkansas		x
California	x	
Colorado	x	
Connecticut		x
Delaware	x	
Florida	x	
Georgia		x
Hawaii	x	
Idaho		x
Illinios	x	
Indiana	x	
Iowa	x	
Kansas		x

State	With Auto Adoption	Without Auto Adoption
Kentucky	x	
Louisiana	x	
Maine		x
Maryland	x	
Massachusetts		x
Michigan		x
Minnesota		x
Mississippi		x
Missouri		x
Montana	x	
Nebraska		x
Nevada		x
New Hampshire		x
New Jersey		x
New Mexico		x
New York	x	
North Carolina	x	
North Dakota		x
Ohio		x
Oklahoma		x
Oregon		x
Pennsylvania		x
Rhode Island	x	
South Carolina	x	
South Dakota		x
Tennessee		x
Texas	x	
Utah	x	
Vermont		x
Virginia		x
Washington	x	
West Virginia		x
Wisconsin	x	
Wyoming		x

SOURCE: FDA, 1990.

SUMMARY OF INDUSTRY COMMENTS

The comments provided by industry generally took the position that FDA has adequately implemented by setting requirements and monitoring compliance of the six provisions of FDCA Section 403 under study. In comments on behalf of Kraft General Foods, Inc., Merrill Thompson suggested that it should be presumed that the FDCA Sections under study and associated FDA regulations are adequate unless demonstrated otherwise (Thompson, 1991).

The Grocery Manufacturers of America (GMA), Inc., made two specific points regarding adequate implementation:

> We have no objection to learning from the states, where they have clearly and significantly improved upon the Federal law and regulations. Where a state cannot demonstrate a unique local condition that requires a unique local solution, but rather has identified a local approach that is superior to the national approach, that approach should indeed be adopted for the entire country. Only in the very rare situation where a state has a unique local condition that requires a unique local solution that is in fact not applicable to the rest of the country should the exemption approach set forth in Section 403(A)(b) be invoked. . . (GMA, 1991).

In its section-by-section evaluation, GMA concluded that current FDA implementation is adequate for all six provisions.

SUMMARY OF CONSUMER INTEREST GROUP COMMENTS

The Center for Science in the Public Interest (CSPI) and other consumer groups provided extensive written comments on the issue of adequate implementation. They concluded that while uniformity is an important goal of NLEA, it is also important that the standards imposed represent the "highest common denominator" of all existing legal requirements, whether Federal, State, or local (CSPI/CNI/CFA/NCL, 1991). This position was echoed by a panel of representatives of both consumer interest groups and government consumer affairs offices who appeared before the Committee. This panel strongly supported the position that the mere existence of a Federal regulation does not in itself constitute adequate implementation and urged that under any circumstance the strictest requirement be adopted as the Federal regulation (Karas, 1991; Rubin, 1991; and Silverglade, 1991).

CSPI and other consumer groups also stressed the important leadership role that States play in responding rapidly to emerging regulatory needs. They provided the following example:

> Another area in which the federal government has not taken the initiative is the issue of "downsizing" or "package shorting," a practice where manufacturers reduce the amount of their product while maintaining the same size container. This area, which relates both to Section 403(d) (misleading containers) and to Section 403(h) (standards of fill), has been the subject of increased public concern as consumers continue to fall prey to this form of economic deception. Foods which have been downsized by manufacturers include canned tuna fish, coffee, tea, cereals, spaghetti sauce and soup mixes. New York is one state which has taken the initiative on this

issue. Currently, a bill has been introduced in New York which would require notice of the package shorting to appear clearly and conspicuously on the principal display panel for at least six months from the date of the package shorting. In contrast, FDA has taken no public action on this issue (CSPI/CNI/CFA/NCL, 1991).

COMMITTEE DELIBERATIONS

Establishing a Foundation for Discussion

The Committee began its deliberation on the issue of adequate implementation by establishing an agreed upon definition of the word *adequate*. The Committee selected Webster's *Third New International Dictionary of the English Language* (unabridged), which provides the following definitions:

Adequate: 1) equal; 2) to make equal or sufficient.

Adequate: 1) equal in size or scope; 2) equal to, proportionate to, or fully sufficient for a specified or implied requirement; narrowly or barely sufficient; no more than satisfactory; 3) legally sufficient, such as is lawfully and reasonably sufficient; 4) fully representative.

Because of the element of subjectivity in the interpretation of several subparts of the definition, the Committee applied its best judgment in concluding that "equal to, proportionate to, or fully sufficient for a specified or implied requirement" best suited its initial needs. The Committee ruled out the remaining options, since they seemed to (1) define physical proportions ("size or scope"); (2) focus on a deficient level of parity ("narrowly or barely"); (3) focus solely on legal criteria; or (4) assume that an agreed upon standard was in place ("fully representative"), and not to embody a relationship that would provide for protection of consumers and public health. The Committee also concluded, however, that it could not apply its chosen definition to carry out its charge without further elaboration.

Discussion of Recommendations to the Committee

Having established a foundation for its discussion, the Committee considered several of the viewpoints summarized earlier in this chapter from Congress, States, the food industry, and consumer groups. The first such view was that it should be presumed that the existing FDCA Sections and any associated FDA regulations adequately implement the purpose of such

Sections. After careful consideration of the NLEA language and the entire *Congressional Record* discussion of NLEA Section 6(b)(1), the Committee rejected this recommendation. It concluded that the existence of Section 6(b)(1) is evidence of the conclusion of Congress that it cannot be presumed that the six FDCA Sections to be studied are being adequately implemented. The Committee also concluded, however, that the absence of an implementing regulation should not lead to an automatic conclusion that implementation is inadequate, although it could raise suspicions. There are two reasons for this conclusion. First, from a legal standpoint, regulations ordinarily are not necessary to implement Federal law. Second, FDA implements policy in ways other than by regulation, and such policy statements deserved consideration by the Committee. However, lack of any formal policy could be troublesome.

A second view, supported especially by States, was that a determination of adequate implementation could not be made without considering whether the statute, regulations, or other implementing policies were being actively and aggressively complied with and enforced. Enforcement was defined as the application of dollar and personnel resources and the use of civil, criminal, or administrative sanctions against violators. States argued that they often established and enforced their own requirements because FDA failed to "enforce" its own statutes, regulations, or other policies. A number of States suggested that Federal implementation would be adequate if only it was well enforced (i.e., Crawford, 1991; Harden, 1991; McClellan, 1991; Niles, 1991).

This second view was particularly troublesome to the Committee. The concerns expressed about the lack of FDA enforcement of policies that were otherwise viewed as adequate in implementing FDCA Section 403 were not without merit. The Committee considered this matter with cognizance of the NLEA provision for State enforcement of Federal law that, in effect, expands the total means available to enforce otherwise adequate provisions. From a pragmatic standpoint, however, the Committee could not ignore the realities of fiscal constraint at all levels of government. If any government agency, Federal, State, or local, has insufficient funding to carry out all of the activities that the agency, or its critics, believe are important to achieve, agency leadership must establish priorities. Historically, such priority setting for resource allocation has been the case, and the Committee is aware of the fact that for many years, FDA's broad enforcement priorities have included health hazards, and filth and related adulteration ahead of economic violations (DHHS, 1991).

From the research it conducted, the Committee could not determine in any conclusive fashion whether or how the States' enforcement of their misbranding statutes differs from that of FDA. Many misbranding charges are settled informally, both at the Federal and State levels. For example, during or after an inspection, a regulator may inform a manufacturer (perhaps orally or in a Warning Letter) that a product appears to be misbranded. Industry may comply (or promise to comply when relabeling), and the matter may end. Alternatively, a formal legal complaint may be filed on behalf of a State or FDA in court, and the complaint then becomes a public document. However, only in instances in which written opinions by a court are collected in a data base system are these decisions easily identified for study. Generally, even these formal agency complaints produce a paper trail that is not easily studied by outside observers unless the matter is of sufficient significance to be reported in the literature and subject to indexing procedures. A reported decision is seldom the result of actions in State trial courts.

The Committee concluded, therefore, that the extent to which FDA enforced the law was a function of national or partisan priorities as established by the elected officials of the executive and/or legislative branches of government. The Committee considered an evaluation of the adequacy of implementation, based on enforcement priority decisions, well beyond its charge, and the view was therefore rejected. The Committee's position was supported by those closely involved in the development of NLEA (Hutt, 1991; Schultz, 1991). The very strong arguments put forward by the proponents of the view (particularly States), that enforcement should be factored into an evaluation of adequacy, however, could not be completely dismissed. The Committee therefore has discussed the issue separately in Chapter 6.

A third view expressed to the Committee was that where more than one implementing requirement existed, whether at the Federal, State, or local level, the strictest requirement should be adopted as the national standard. In considering this question, the Committee was confronted with the problem of defining *strictness*. In many cases, the differences between Federal and State requirements were small, and their relative significance was not readily apparent. For example, in the case of canned oysters, FDA and a number of States have set standards for fill of container that are different, with no readily apparent reason for the differences. In other instances, the Committee was concerned that unnecessarily strict requirements had been established to protect local industries rather than the public. In the final analysis, the Committee concluded that, absent specific justification, the strictest requirement was not always the best for national implementation and, therefore, rejected this view. An additional reason to reject this view was that it could mean that all FDA requirements were inadequate without more stringent standards.

The Committee chose instead to base its conclusions on a consideration of its own criteria.

Sources Other Than Regulations for Determining
Adequacy of FDA Implementation

Beyond regulations, a tremendous variety of written materials analyze, interpret, and discuss FDA's view of its statutory mandate. These documents include proposed regulations, preambles to proposed and final regulations, Compliance Policy Guides, guidelines, advisory opinions, letters to the regulated industry, Regulatory and Notice of Adverse Findings letters (both now called Warning Letters), records of court actions, speeches, press releases, and speeches given by FDA officials. At one time or another, FDA has used all of these materials as a way of implementing the law. The Committee concluded, however, that it would be impractical to examine all of them because (1) ensuring that all relevant documents had been discovered would be difficult, (2) all of these documents might not offer consistent advice, (3) no practical indexes or other means for retrieval exist except for hand searching, and (4) many of these mechanisms do not legally bind the agency. Accordingly, the Committee decided to examine only those mechanisms that FDA agrees bind it to a particular position.

FDA has outlined the procedure that the public may use to seek a formal advisory opinion on the agency's view of the laws it administers (21 CFR §10.85). According to FDA, an advisory opinion represents the formal position of the agency on a matter; except in unusual situations that involve an immediate and significant danger to health, the agency is obligated to act in accordance with the opinion until it is amended or revoked [21 CFR §10.85(e)]. In addition to advisory opinions issued through the procedure outlined in 21 CFR §10.85, FDA has also identified in that section a number of other documents to which it accords the status of formal advisory opinions (unless they are subsequently repudiated by FDA or overruled by a court):

1. Any portion of a *Federal Register* notice other than the text of a proposed or final regulation, for example, a notice to manufacturers or a preamble to a proposed or final regulation.
2. Trade Correspondence (TC Nos. 1 through 431, and 1A through 8A) issued by FDA between 1938 and 1946.
3. Compliance policy guides issued by FDA beginning in 1968 and codified in the Compliance Policy Guides manual.

4. Other documents specifically identified as advisory opinions, for example, advisory opinions on the performance standard for diagnostic x-ray systems, issued before July 1, 1975, and filed in a permanent public file for prior advisory opinions maintained by the Freedom of Information staff.
5. Guidelines issued by FDA under 21 CFR 10.90(b), which establishes the procedure for the issuance of guidelines [21 CFR 10.85 (d)].

Since FDA has publicly agreed to bind itself by these materials, it seems fair to view them as the agency's official implementation of the statute. The Committee judged that this approach provided ample material with which to work and perform its task.

A second consideration for the Committee was the impact of the provisions of FDCA Sections 403(a)(1), 403(e), and 403(i)(2) on the adequacy of FDA implementation when coupled with the requirements of the six provisions that are the subject of this study. Because FDA can bring charges in cases of violation of FDCA under more than one section, the Committee concluded that this interrelationship could not be ignored. Indeed, when the Committee reviewed the enforcement history of regulatory actions taken by FDA, it invariably encountered charges under multiple sections of FDCA.

For example, FDCA Section 403(a)(1) states that a food will be deemed to be misbranded if its labeling is false or misleading in any particular. A food in package form is considered misbranded under FDCA Section 403(e) unless it bears a label containing (1) the name and place of business of the manufacturer, packer, or distributor; and (2) an accurate statement of quantity of contents. FDCA Section 403(i)(2) raises another misbranding issue: in cases in which a food is fabricated from two or more ingredients, the label must bear the common or usual name of each such ingredient (with limited exceptions), or the product will be considered misbranded. These three sections affected the Committee's review of the adequacy of implementation of FDCA Sections 403(b) [food offered for sale under the name of another food], and 403(i)(1) [common or usual name]. The Committee, however, was careful not to attribute greater significance to the requirements of FDCA Sections 403(a)(1), 403(e), and 403(i)(2) than was appropriate for the study. On the other hand, these three sections were not ignored when the Committee considered the overall ability of FDA to implement an adequate food labeling regulatory program.

Two other components of Federal regulations that could be considered in adequate implementation are compliance and enforcement. Compliance would address the issue of the extent to which manufacturers have met the provisions of the laws and regulations, i.e. the degree to which food labels in the marketplace comply with the Federal labeling requirements. An evaluation of enforcement would address the extent to which FDA has pursued manufacturers that market products with labels that do not meet the Federal requirements. With regard to compliance as a measure of adequate implementation, this criterion was considered to be important because it represents the effectiveness of existing requirements to fulfill the Congressional mandate of FDCA. However, this issue was not mentioned as a criterion in either the provisions of NLEA, or the Congressional debate on the subject. In addition, the Committee received no information on compliance from its requests to FDA and the States. Anecdotal cases of violations were cited in discussions with State officials, but no comprehensive record of noncompliance was available for the Committee's use. Although the Committee recognized the critical importance of compliance to an evaluation of adequate implementation, the absence of compliance data required the Committee to omit inclusion of compliance as a criteria for determining adequacy of implementation of the six provisions of FDCA Section 403 under study.

The Committee also considered the question of whether FDA's enforcement of existing laws and regulations should be a criterion for evaluating the adequacy of implementation of the six provisions of FDCA Section 403. To determine the intent of Congress on whether enforcement was an issue for the Committee's consideration, it reviewed the provisions of NLEA and the Congressional record debate on the issue and discussed the question with a number of individuals familiar with the course of the Act's development. No evidence was presented to the Committee which would indicate that enforcement was an anticipated criterion for determining adequacy of implementation. While the Committee believed that the issue of enforcement was important in terms of evaluating the agency's implementation record, it also recognized that FDA's enforcement record is significantly influenced by resources available (adequate manpower and funding) and the political will at given points in time. Therefore, the Committee chose not to include enforcement as a criterion for adequate implementation. However, because enforcement was considered to be an important issue for the future, the issue is addressed at considerable length later in the report.

State Regulations as an Indicator of Adequacy of FDA Implementation

The two most frequently cited justifications for State regulation were that (1) States provide an avenue by which new and innovative regulatory approaches can be developed and tested prior to adoption at the Federal level, and (2) States have often found it necessary to regulate in the absence of Federal leadership. Without passing judgment on the merits of these arguments, the Committee concluded that its review of State laws and regulations could provide one measure of the adequacy of Federal implementation. Therefore, in reviewing State laws and regulations, the Committee was sensitive to the following indicators:

1. The frequency with which different States regulated a practice regardless of any FDA regulation.
2. The regulation by one or more States of a matter considered by the Committee to be of national importance and/or prominence.
3. The regulation by a State of a matter of strictly local significance to both consumers and industry.
4. The regulation by a State of a matter resulting in the economic protection of the industry, without consumer benefit.

The basis for the review of State requirements was the tasks defined in the proposed plan of action presented by the Institute of Medicine (IOM). In broader terms, the Committee was required to carry out the following tasks:

1. Identify existing State/local laws with provisions applicable to food labeling reform efforts currently being undertaken by FDA as related to FDCA Sections 403(b), 403(d), 403(f), 403(h), 403(i)(1), and 403(k).
2. Summarize those State/local laws with relevant provisions and, if supporting data are provided by State/local regulators, consider the public health issues that prompted the development of the provisions.
3. Assess the extent to which each of the six Sections of FDCA is being implemented; in addition, to the extent required by the six Sections of FDCA, evaluate existing data on the effect on public health and nutrition of preempting applicable State/local laws.
4. Hold at least one open meeting to permit representatives of State/local governments and other interested persons to submit information relative to State/local laws and regulations for food labeling and comment on the adequacy of Federal implementation of the six relevant Sections of the FDCA.
5. Identify, prioritize, and recommend those provisions that should be given consideration by FDA in its food labeling reform efforts.

One definitional problem had a significant impact on the Committee's review of State requirements and preemption determinations. Under NLEA,

State standards of identity that are different from Federal standards of identity were preempted on the date NLEA was enacted (November 8, 1990). However, a State statute or regulation setting forth a common or usual name for a food that is not identical to the requirements of FDCA Section 403(i)(1) is not immediately preempted but subject to review after the conclusion of this study. If preemption occurs, it will become effective November 8, 1992. However, regulatory areas of concern to the States cannot easily be categorized. Therefore, it is difficult to determine from a legal point of view whether State requirements are (1) "standards of identity" that are different from Federal standard, and thus already preempted by NLEA; (2) "standards of identity" in cases in which no Federal standards exist and therefore may not be preempted; or (3) "common or usual names" that are different from Federal standards, not yet preempted, and thus subject to the Committee's review for determination of the adequacy of Federal requirements.

The Committee decided that it could not distinguish in any principled way among these three categories of misbranding and therefore it would view its own jurisdiction broadly. If it was reasonable to consider that the State regulation fell within the purview of the Committee's jurisdiction, it was treated as a matter for study. Because the conclusions of the Committee are only recommendations to FDA about which State requirements it should consider embracing, the Committee felt that it would be appropriate in its categorization of State requirements to take the broader rather than the narrower approach to the interpretation of NLEA.

DEVELOPING THE COMMITTEE'S CRITERIA

In carrying out its charge, the Committee evaluated the adequacy of FDA's implementation of the six provisions of FDCA Section 403 in the following manner. First, it applied the principles developed through its own deliberative process:

1. The definition of *adequate* as "equal to, proportionate to, or fully sufficient for a specified or implied requirement" was used as a foundation for decisions.
2. The intent of any section and any regulation, as interpreted by the Committee, was a consideration, including, as appropriate, a consideration of the impact of Sections 403(a)(1), 403(e), and 403(i)(2) when used in conjunction with the six provisions that are the subject of the study.

3. The absence of an FDA implementing regulation would not lead to an automatic conclusion that implementation was inadequate.
4. The level of enforcement would not be a consideration in determining adequacy of implementation.
5. The strictest requirement, whether Federal, State, or local, would not automatically be recommended for adoption as the national standard.
6. The Committee limited its study of the six FDCA sections to any implementing regulations for which rulemaking had been completed and published advisory opinions as defined in 21 CFR §10.85.
7. In reviewing State and local requirements and their relationship to the six provisions of FDCA under study, the Committee viewed its own jurisdiction broadly to ensure a fair, balanced review of the materials provided by State and local officials and other interested persons.

Second, the Committee reviewed and evaluated all State requirements it had assembled against the tasks defined in the IOM Proposed Plan of Action described earlier in this chapter.

Third, the Committee categorized the State requirements according to the following criteria:

1. An adequate Federal requirement exists on the issue (the field is thus occupied).
2. The agency has not adequately implemented the Act in the area of concern represented by the State requirement. Such a conclusion would be based on the requirement's national importance, its national prominence as indicated by the frequency of attention to the issue by the States, and/or the lack of an existing Federal regulation.
3. The State requirement meets a demonstrated local need.
4. The State requirement provides only economic protection to the industry, is without consumer benefit, and/or has no other redeeming virtue.

As part of its consideration of adequacy, the Committee has suggested the adoption of State requirements by FDA that might otherwise be preempted if, in its judgment, those requirements clearly provide special benefit to the consumer. To the extent possible, it has also established priorities among the candidates under criteria 2 and 3 above. Under this approach, the Committee left to FDA the legal determination of whether certain State requirements (statutes and/or regulations) were "definitions and standards" or "common or usual names," and the steps necessary under NLEA regarding their preemption. The results of the review and evaluation process outlined above and the Committee's categorization of State requirements are discussed in the next chapter.

REFERENCES

AFDO (Association of Food and Drug Officials). 1991. Letter to the Committee on State Food Labeling, Food and Nutrition Board, Institute of Medicine, Washington, D.C. July 1.

Crawford, B., Florida Department of Agriculture and Consumer Services. 1991. Letter to the Committee on State Food Labeling, Food and Nutrition Board, Institute of Medicine, Washington, D.C. May 30.

CSPI/CNI/CFA/NCL (Center for Science in the Public Interest, Community Nutrition Institute, Consumer Federation of America, and the National Consumers League). 1991. Statement of Sharon Lindan, Assistant Director for Legal Affairs, CSPI, on behalf of CSPI/CNI/CFA/NCL at the Public Meeting of the Committee on State Food Labeling, Food and Nutrition Board, Institute of Medicine, Washington, D.C. May 30.

DHHS (Department of Health and Human Services). 1991. Final Report of the Advisory Committee on the Food and Drug Administration. Washington, D.C.: Government Printing Office.

FDA (Food and Drug Administration). 1972. Nonstandardized Foods; Proposed Common or Usual Names. Fed. Reg. 37:12327; June 22.

FDA (Food and Drug Administration). 1973. Common or Usual Names for Nonstandardized Foods. Final Rule. Fed. Reg. 38:6964–6967; March 14.

FDA (Food and Drug Administration). 1979. Administrative Practice and Procedures. Final Rule. Fed. Reg. 44:22318–22370; April 13.

FDA (Food and Drug Administration). 1981. Reorganizational/Location Changes. Final Rule. 46 Fed. Reg. 8454-8462; January 27.

FDA (Food and Drug Administration). 1990. State Law Data: 1990. Rockville, Md.: FDA.

FDA (Food and Drug Administration). 1991. State Petitions Requesting Exemption from Federal Preemption. Proposed Rule. Fed. Reg. 56:60528-60534; Nov. 27.

GMA (Grocery Manufacturers of America). 1991. Statement of Sherwin Gardner, Vice President, Science and Technology, GMA, at the Public Meeting of the Committee on State Food Labeling, Food and Nutrition Board, Institute of Medicine, Washington, D.C. May 30.

Hamilton, R.W. 1972. Procedures for the adoption of rules of general application: The need for procedural innovation in administrative rulemaking. Calif. Law Rev. 60:1276–1337.

Harden, B., Maryland Department of Health and Mental Hygiene. 1991. Letter to the Committee on State Food Labeling, Food and Nutrition Board, Institute of Medicine, Washington, D.C. June 6.

Hutt, P.B., 1973. Philosophy of regulation under the Federal Food, Drug, and Cosmetic Act. Food Drug Cosmetic Law J. 28:177–188.

Hutt, P.B. 1991. Presentation by Peter Barton Hutt, Partner, Covington and Burling, before the Committee on State Food Labeling, Food and Nutrition Board, Institute of Medicine, Washington, D.C. May 29.

Hutt, P.B., and R.A. Merrill. 1991. Food and Drug Law: Cases and Materials. 2nd ed. Westbury, N.Y.: The Foundation Press.

Karas, A. 1991. Presentation by Amy Karas, New York Department of Consumer Affairs, before the Committee on State Food Labeling, Food and Nutrition Board, Institute of Medicine, Washington, D.C. July 29.

Levinson, B.D. c. 1952. Regulations Under the Federal Food, Drug, and Cosmetic Act. Washington, D.C.: Federal Security Agency.

McClellan, D., Utah Department of Agriculture. 1991. Letter to the Committee on State Food Labeling, Food and Nutrition Board, Institute of Medicine, Washington, D.C. July 8.

Mintz, B.W., and N.G. Miller. 1991. A Guide to Federal Agency Rulemaking. Washington, D.C.: Administrative Conference of the United States.

Niles, R., Georgia Department of Agriculture. 1991. Letter to the Committee on State Food Labeling, Food and Nutrition Board, Institute of Medicine, Washington, D.C. June 17.

Pfeifer, E.M. 1984. 1984 Enforcement. Pp. 72–113 in Seventy-fifth Anniversary Commemorative Volume of Food and Drug Law. Washington, D.C.: Food and Drug Law Institute.

Rubin, B. 1991. Presentation by Barry Rubin, General Counsel, The Advocacy Institute, before the Committee on State Food Labeling, Food and Nutrition Board, Institute of Medicine, Washington, D.C. July 29.

Schultz, W. 1991. Presentation by William Schultz, Counsel, Subcommittee on Health and Environment, House Committee on Energy and Commerce, U.S. Congress, before the Committee on State Food Labeling, Food and Nutrition Board, Institute of Medicine, Washington, D.C. July 30.

Silverglade, B. 1991. Presentation by Bruce Silverglade, Director of Legal Affairs, Center for Science in the Public Interest, before the Committee on State Food Labeling, Food and Nutrition Board, Institute of Medicine, Washington, D.C. July 29.

State Attorneys General. 1991. Statement of Attorneys General of California, Iowa, Minnesota, Missouri, New York, Texas, and Wisconsin to the Committee on State Food Labeling, Food and Nutrition Board, Institute of Medicine, Washington, D.C. May 30.

Thompson, M.S., Special Counsel, Arnold & Porter. 1991. Letter to the Committee on State Food Labeling, Food and Nutrition Board, Institute of Medicine, Washington, D.C. May 14.

U.S. Congress, House. 1990. Nutrition Labeling and Education Act of 1990. Move to suspend the rules and pass the bill (H.R. 3562). Congressional Record-House, H5836-H5845.

WHC (White House Conference on Food, Nutrition, and Health). 1969. Final Report. Washington, D.C.: Government Printing Office.

5

Comparison and Analysis of Federal and State Food Labeling Requirements

The Committee collected information from the sources outlined in Chapters 2 and 4, first categorizing it according to the six provisions of the Federal Food, Drug, and Cosmetic Act (FDCA) under study and then analyzing it. This chapter presents the analysis of those data with conclusions and recommendations related to the criteria outlined in Chapter 4. The discussion of the six provisions of FDCA Section 403 under study covers current Federal legal authority and regulations, the relationship of provisions to other FDCA misbranding sections and related Federal laws, a review of State and available local statutes, a summary of State, industry and consumer perspectives, and the Committee's conclusions.

COMPLEXITY OF THE ANALYSIS AND COVERAGE

The charge to the Committee was to study State and local food labeling requirements that were not identical to FDCA Sections 403(b), 403(d), 403(f), 403(h), 403(i)(1), and 403(k), as identified in Section 6 of the Nutrition Labeling and Education Act (NLEA). Although this mandate initially appeared straightforward, the nature of the laws and regulations involved and the ambiguities present in NLEA made the Committee's fulfillment of its mandate a complex task.

First, it was not possible in all cases to determine whether a particular State or local food labeling law and/or regulation was similar to one of the specific FDCA sections under study. In numerous instances, State laws and regulations did not address the specific misbranding issues dealt with in the six study provisions. In other cases, State requirements appeared both to require labeling "of the type" regulated under one or more of the six provisions of FDCA Section 403 under study and be either a standard of identity or analogous to other FDCA provisions (e.g., imitation, ingredient labeling) for which automatic preemption applied. Finally, some State requirements appeared to be related to both FDCA misbranding provisions, subject to NLEA, and adulteration sections, which are excluded from consideration.

Because many State requirements did not fall neatly into only one of the six study provisions, the Committee used its best judgment to classify and review State food labeling requirements under the provision it considered most appropriate. It did not review labeling issues that were clearly outside its charge (e.g., origin labeling, which is regulated by the U.S. Customs Service and the Federal Trade Commission). Based on the legislative history and text of NLEA, the Committee also excluded from its deliberations concerns related to food safety, grading, kosher, organic, natural, and open-date labeling. In addition, the Committee excluded any analysis of emerging State and local regulatory issues (e.g., environmental "green" labeling), although it believes some of these issues deserve consideration by the Food and Drug Administration (FDA; see Chapter 6).

It was not surprising to the Committee that many State food labeling requirements fit into multiple provisions of FDCA Section 403 because provisions of the Act itself overlap considerably. For example, a requirement that a food bearing a certain name contain a prescribed amount of a particular food constituent may seem to prescribe a standard of identity at the same time that it constitutes a common or usual name requirement.

If the Committee's charge had been only to classify a State food labeling requirement as parallel to one rather than another of the six provisions of FDCA Section 403 under study, which Section was chosen would be of little concern because the implications for preemption would be identical. The Committee recognized, however, that these FDCA provisions have developed over time, beginning with those whose forerunners were contained in the Pure Food and Drugs Act of 1906 [PFDA; i.e., Section 403(b)] and they have been modified by addition rather than by consolidation. Further, from a practical standpoint, it is common FDA enforcement practice to charge violators with violation of multiple FDCA sections. These factors made the Committee's review of FDA requirements and case histories more difficult. However, as discussed earlier, the Committee decided to view its own task broadly: for example, if it was reasonable to view a State regulation as a common or usual name requirement (even if a court might later determine it to be a standard of identity), it was treated as a matter for study by the Committee. Because it was to make recommendations to FDA about which State requirements it should consider adopting, the Committee felt that it would be entirely appropriate to take the broader rather than the narrower approach. To illustrate this view, Appendix H contains a summary of State requirements for names of frequently cited food commodities. The issue is addressed further in the discussion of FDCA Section 403(i)(1) (common or usual names).

Finally, the Committee reached all but a very few of its conclusions through consensus. There were several instances in which strongly held views of individual members kept the Committee from reaching complete agreement. When this occurred, the text expresses both views. The Committee's final conclusions on these matters reflect the view of a majority of its members.

FOOD UNDER THE NAME OF ANOTHER FOOD—SECTION 403(b)

FDCA Section 403(b) states that a food is misbranded "if it is offered for sale under the name of another food."

Federal Requirements

Section 403(b) is characterized as a general provision of FDCA Section 403, derived from the 1906 PFDA. Among other requirements, the 1906 Act provided that a food shall not be deemed to be misbranded

in the case of mixtures or compounds which may be now or from time to time hereafter known as articles of food, under their own distinctive names, and not an imitation of or offered for sale under the distinctive name of another article, if the name be accompanied on the same label or brand with a statement of the place where said article has been manufactured or produced.

Section 403(b) was a noncontroversial holdover from the 1906 Act that represents a generalized statement of the type of requirement that has been expanded in more specific provisions of FDCA Sections 403(g) and (i)(1). The distinction between FDCA Section 403(i)(1) [common or usual names], and Section 403(b) is ambiguous. When FDA has charged manufacturers with violations of FDCA Section 403(b), it has usually done so together with other provisions of FDCA Section 403. The use of multiple sections of FDCA in bringing legal actions reflects, among other things, the duplication among the several misbranding provisions. Section 403(b) also protects against some of the same concerns as those addressed in FDCA Section 402, the economic adulteration provision. The intent of FDCA Section 403(b) is to prohibit the use of misleading names of foods when there is no common or usual name or definition and standard of identity for a food. (For example, a food cannot be labeled as crabmeat if it does not contain crabmeat or contains other fish meat without appropriate labeling.)

The case most frequently cited as an example in which FDA relied exclusively on the prohibition basic to Section 403(b) involves apple cider vinegar, brought under the provisions of the 1906 Act. In this action, the government prevailed in its contention that vinegar produced from dehydrated apples and water was not "apple cider vinegar." The court ruled that cider is the expressed juice of apples, both popularly and generally known as such, and the product made from dehydrated apples and water did not represent "apple cider vinegar" *U.S. v. 95 Barrels*, 265 U.S. 438, 44 S.Ct. 529 (1924).

Hutt and Merrill (1991) point out the close relationship between FDCA Sections 403(b) and 402(b):

> Like the economic adulteration provisions, which are essentially designed to prevent the marketing of debased foods, section 403(b) requires a court to identify a standard against which to compare the product involved, *i.e.,* the "other" food that the seized product is charged with imitating. The need for a standard of comparison is common to statutory as well as common law theories that are concerned primarily with "passing off" offenses (p. 53).

The need for a standard of comparison was reinforced by the Bireley's orange beverage case [*U.S. v. 88 Cases*, 187 F.2d 967 (3d Cir. 1951)], an economic adulteration case. In that case, the government failed to prevail because the product could not be condemned unless there was a confusion with a defined superior product; it was not sufficient for consumers merely to consider that the drink contained more orange than it did. A violation of Section 403(b) could not be found "without a finding that a marketable inferior product is likely to be confused with a specified superior counterpart" (Hutt and Merrill, 1991). FDA has reiterated the language of FDCA Section 403(b) at 21 CFR §101.18(a), but it has not expanded or further elaborated on its meaning.

FDA has also exempted selected foods from the general labeling requirements, including Section 403(b). Individually wrapped pieces of candy and other confectionery of less than 0.5 ounce per package are exempt from labeling requirements when the container in which they are shipped is in compliance [21 CFR §1.24(a)(4)]. In addition, eggs packaged in cartons of a dozen that can be divided into two six-egg containers are exempt if the original carton is adequately labeled, even though one of the resulting six-egg containers would not be in compliance [21 CFR 1.24(a)(9)(i)].

In the 1970s, FDA began formally to establish common or usual names for nonstandardized foods as an alternative to the procedurally burdensome process of establishing standards of identity for foods. The protection offered by this process overlaps considerably with FDCA Section 403(b). Today, for example, there is a common or usual name regulation for diluted orange juice beverage (21 CFR §102.32). Part 102 also establishes common or usual names for peanut spreads (21 CFR §102.23) and potato chips made from dried potatoes (21 CFR §102.41), as well as a variety of nonstandardized fish and other products.

State Requirements

Statements received by the Committee from States focused on enforcement of FDCA Section 403(b). For example, in his letter to the Committee, Ray Niles, Assistant Director of the Consumer Protection Division, Georgia Department of Agriculture, stated that:

> We feel that the FDCA, as well as title 21 CFR, adequately addresses misbranding of food (name of food under the name of the other), but we also feel there is no enforcement being taken in that area. As an example, soybean "cheese" is sold as cheese. The CFR's define cheese and exclude soybeans. More enforcement action would halt this practice. Another more glaring example of food sold under the name of another food is the failure of FDA to address well or municipal waters sold as "spring water" (Niles, 1991a).

Industry Perspective

Industry comments reflect the same concerns as those of the States regarding FDCA Section 403(b) and revolve around the use of misleading or fraudulent names for nonstandardized foods. It has been suggested that FDA recently has been less vigorous than in the past in addressing the naming of new foods and the agency should return to its policy of the 1970s by which it established such names. The Grocery Manufacturers of America (GMA) urged the Committee "to review this matter and to recommend that FDA reestablish the policy regarding common or usual names for nonstandardized food that the agency pursued at that time" (GMA, 1991).

Consumer Perspective

Consumer views of FDCA Section 403(b) coincide with those of the States and industry. Their concern is that the label properly identify the exact nature of the product sold (CSPI/CNI/CFA/NCL, 1991).

Conclusions

The Committee perceived no major difference among the views of States, industry, and consumer groups on FDA implementation of FDCA Section 403(b), which was perceived as adequate. However, all parties were concerned with FDA's poor enforcement of current requirements or slow establishment of additional common or usual names [FDCA Section 403(i)(1)]. As discussed in Chapter 4, the Committee chose not to include enforcement as a measurement of adequate implementation but concurs with the concerns of these groups related to the establishment of common or usual names (see discussion later in this chapter).

Based on its analysis and criteria, the Committee concludes that FDCA Section 403(b) has been adequately implemented. The Committee further concludes that State requirements related to FDCA Section 403(b) are candidates for preemption. To promote the development and introduction of new foods, however, the Committee suggests that FDA pursue more aggressively the regulatory options that will allow the formal naming of new nonstandardized foods. Additionally, as part of its annual consideration of administrative revisions to FDCA, the Committee suggests that FDA consider consolidation of the objective of FDCA Section 403(b) with that of FDCA Section 403(i)(1).

CONTAINER FILL AND DECEPTIVE PACKAGING—SECTION 403(d)

FDCA Section 403(d) states that a food is misbranded "if its container is so made, formed, or filled as to be misleading."

Federal Requirements

From the beginning of deliberations to revise PFDA in 1933, a major legislative goal was to provide stronger regulation to prevent slack fill and deceptive packaging. Throughout the legislative consideration, the "so made, formed, or filled" language was understood to ban "deceptive or slack filled containers." The term "slack fill" refers to the partial filling of a package, even though the actual net quantity of the contents is accurately labeled. The term "deceptive packaging" refers to the use of a container that is made to appear to have a larger amount of the product than is actually in the container, even though the part of the container designed to hold the product is completely filled and the net quantity of the contents is accurately stated. Deceptive packaging may occur by use of false bottoms, thick side walls, or other structural techniques.

The "so made, formed, or filled" provisions of FDCA combined the specific concept of slack fill, which applies only to the level of fill in the immediate product container, and the general concept of deceptive packaging, which applies broadly to all aspects of product packaging. During the five years of Congressional debate on this issue, the language for this section remained unchanged: the term "filled" referred to the problem of slack fill, while the terms "made" and "formed" referred to other kinds of deceptive packaging (Hutt, 1987).

Hutt (1987) also provides a description of the implementation of the slack fill and deceptive packaging provisions in FDCA Section 403(d). FDA has the authority under FDCA Section 401 to establish a specific standard for fill of container for particular food commodities and thus prohibit by regulation any nonfunctional slack fill. The agency, in its discretion, however, has determined that this is not a practical way to implement the Congressional policy embodied in FDCA Section 403(d) for all food (although it has done so in many standards of identity). FDA has also decided not to use its discretionary authority to promulgate general regulations governing slack fill under Section 403(d). The agency's argument in both instances is that it is not cost-effective to establish detailed regulations governing nonfunctional slack fill for all food products or specific food product classes; to make any such regulations realistic and supportable would require consideration of the specific characteristics of each of the individual food commodities and types of packaging involved. FDA considers the expenditure of agency resources that would be needed for such an extensive, complex effort highly disproportionate to the size of any problem being encountered in the marketplace. To combat misleading packaging, however, the agency has at its disposal the minimum basic label requirements, such as net weight of container, set forth under FDCA Section 403(e).

To date, formal FDA implementation of FDCA Section 403(d) has been limited to a few court cases, all of which the agency lost. It may be that FDA has been successful in pursuing violations that have not resulted in reported decisions by courts; for example, violators may have become compliant before court action was necessary (Hutt, 1987). FDA Trade Correspondence (TC) offers historical evidence of agency rulings regarding specific concerns about slack fill. One such piece of correspondence, dated March 14, 1940, states that "*gelatin dessert packages* should be redesigned to avoid *slack filling* and consequent deception" (TC-161); correspondence dated August 20, 1940, notes that " [g]elatin dessert packages, to avoid charge of deception, should provide maximum fill with minimum of unavoidable unoccupied space" (TC-318). The standard adopted in the Arden Assorted Candy Drops case, *U.S. v. 116 Boxes*, 80 F.Supp. 911, 913 (D.Mass.1948), was that the court should consider whether the container is "likely to mislead the ordinary purchaser of this type of merchandise, not one who was particularly attentive or prudent." In a case involving slack filled candy bars, *U.S. v. Caraldo*, 157 F.2d 802, 804 (1st Cir.1946), the court held that there is no "hard and fast rule as to what would constitute slack-filling," and, therefore, it is a question of fact for the district court to decide. Further, as another court ruled, even if the container may deceive the purchaser into thinking it contains more than it does, the filling of the container may be "justified by considerations of safety" and reasonable in light of possible alternatives. However, the court noted as an example that although "some padding is obviously necessary in egg crates to safeguard the eggs, . . . a 2-inch cotton cushion between each of the eggs would not be justified, even though such padding would serve fully the ends of safety," *U.S. v. 174 Cases (Delson Thin Mints)*, 287 F.2d 246, 248 (3d. Cir. 1961).

Related Sections of Law

There is some degree of overlap between the wording of FDCA Sections 403(d) and 403(h), both of which address concerns related to fill of container. As a result, confusion can arise in the interpretation of Section 403(d) by the casual reader. Section 403(d) establishes the general provision that a food shall be deemed to be misbranded "if its container is so made, formed, or filled as to be misleading." On the other hand, FDCA Section 403(h)(2) must be read in context with FDCA Section 401, which authorizes FDA to establish by regulation specific criteria for evaluating the fill of container for certain food products. FDCA Section 403(h)(2) requires that a product be labeled as substandard if it fails to meet the FDCA Section 401 standard. This latter requirement is discussed more fully under FDCA Section 403(h)(2).

In addition to the provisions of FDCA, the Federal Fair Packaging and Labeling Act of 1966 (FPLA) provided FDA with additional rulemaking authority [FPLA Section 5(c)(4)] to define nonfunctional slack fill on a commodity-by-commodity basis. To date, FDA has not chosen to promulgate regulations. It is important to note that California believed there is a need for additional consumer protection in this area and has adopted a nonfunctional slack fill provision identical to the language of FPLA (Cal. Bus. & Prof. Code §12606).

State Requirements

Several State Attorneys General (1991) have suggested that States often take the lead in responding to the public's needs locally in advance of any Federal response. They cited the example of regulation of misleading package containers as an instance in which they believed States were providing such leadership. Some States have enacted laws or promulgated regulations that indicate a different resolution of container fill and deceptive packaging policy issues from that of FDA.

Representatives from the Florida Department of Agriculture and Consumer Services (FDACS) cited several examples of commercially available food products that in their opinion are deceptively packaged (Woodward, 1991). In one case, a manufacturer made two varieties of single-serving packets of powdered hot beverage mix. The variety that was called "light" contained 40 percent less product by weight, but the size of the envelopes and external package for both varieties were the same. FDACS considers Federal action on deceptive packaging inadequate, especially for products in opaque containers. Likewise, Michigan expressed a need for greater clarity of FDA policies relative to container fill and deceptive packaging.

Some State and local jurisdictions have also addressed the matter of "downsizing" of products or "package shorting," the practice of reducing the amount of product in a package while maintaining the same size container. Downsizing is considered an issue of deceptive packaging rather than slack fill. Examples of foods that have been alleged to be downsized by manufacturers include canned tuna fish, coffee, tea, cereals, spaghetti sauce, and soup mixes. New York recently introduced legislation that would require notice of the package change to appear clearly and conspicuously on the principal display panel for at least 6 months from the date the downsizing occurs (AFDO, 1991; Lindan, 1991). In contrast, no Federal regulations deal with the practice of downsizing.

The following list outlines State labeling requirements "of the type" represented by FDCA Section 403(d):

Alabama has enacted specific rules for "fill" of food packages (Ala. Ag. Rule no. 80-1-22-.10).

Alaska requires that "a fisheries product is misbranded if . . . its container is made, formed, or filled in a manner that is misleading . . ." (Alaska Stat. §18-34.160).

California prohibits nonfunctional slack fill of containers unless it is (a) necessary to protect the contents of the package or (b) required by the machines used to pack the contents in such packages (Cal. Health & Safety Code §26437). A second California requirement for deceptive packaging which prohibits all nonfunctional slack fill packaging is discussed below (Cal. Bus. & Prof. Code §12606).

Connecticut requirements prohibit deceptive packaging or filling of the container by requiring that no commodity in package form shall be wrapped or in a container that is formed or filled to mislead the purchaser as to the quantity or the quality of the contents of the package (Conn. Gen. Stat. §42-115m). Furthermore, the contents of a container shall not fall below such reasonable standard of fill as may have been prescribed for the commodity in question by the Commissioner of Consumer Affairs.

Minnesota has established tolerances and variations from the quantity of contents marked on packages. The only allowable discrepancies are those owing to (1) unavoidable errors when weighing the product in compliance with good commercial practices, (2) differences in capacities of bottles and similar containers resulting from unavoidable manufacturing difficulties, or (3) atmospheric conditions (Minn. R. §1550.0480).

New Jersey has introduced a State bill which requires that consumers must receive clear and conspicuous label notice for at least six months in instances in which the net weight, measure, or quantity of food in a package has been reduced without a substantial change in packaging (N.J. Bill 4880, pending).

Washington requires that any slack filled container shall be conspicuously marked "slack filled" (Wash. Rev. Code §69.28.100).

The activities in California to regulate misleading packaging deserve further discussion because the State has chosen to implement FPLA requirements that go beyond FDA requirements. The California Attorney General interpreted the State's slack fill provision as not requiring proof that the slack fill is misleading or deceptive and prohibiting any unoccupied space in cases in which the immediate container is enclosed within an outer retail package (e.g., a bottle in a cardboard carton). In *Hobby Industry Association of America, Inc. v. Younger,* 101 Cal. App. 3d 358, 161 Cal. Rptr. 601 (1980), the court upheld the position of the California Attorney General.

As so interpreted, this California provision (Cal. Bus. & Prof. Code §12606) is clearly "of the type" covered by Section 403(d), because both address slack fill. The interpretation of Section 12606 appears not to be identical to the Federal interpretation, however, because it prohibits all "nonfunctional slack fill packaging whether or not there is other proof of deception or fraud." The language of FPLA was adopted as the standard by California in developing its State statute.

By prohibiting what it considers to be inherently misleading slack fill, California has been particularly aggressive in adopting a unique approach that differs from that of FDA and other States. It may be that other States have not identified this issue as a problem worthy of independent legislative action (GMA, 1991). As the Assistant Director of the Consumer Protection Division of the Georgia Department of Agriculture stated, "We have not encountered problems with container fill and deceptive packaging. If we do, we feel the FDCA is more than adequate if enforced. Sections 101.18 and 101.105 of Title 21 CFR adequately deal with this, but again, lack enforcement" (Niles, 1991a).

However, in the view of the State Attorneys General and many other State officials, until such time as FDA promulgates regulations to interpret this section of FDCA, statutes such as California Business and Professions Code Section 12606 and any State statutes dealing with downsizing should prevail (State Attorneys General, 1991).

Industry Perspective

GMA supports the decision of FDA not to promulgate regulations pertaining to FDCA Section 403(d). The Association's comment to the Committee was that "that determination should stand as the national approach to the matter" (GMA, 1991).

A representative of the National Frozen Pizza Institute (NFPI) indicated that, despite FDA's failure to establish violations of FDCA Section 403(d) through litigation, the Institute also believes that FDA has adequately implemented this provision. Support for this argument comes from the fact that the Act requires the net weight statement to appear on every package and, in many cases, FDA has established specific product standards of fill (NFPI, 1991). This same view was held by a representative speaking on behalf of the Quaker Oats Company and Schreiber Foods, Inc. (Quaker Oats and Schreiber Foods, 1991).

Consumer Perspective

Consumer groups stated that the absence of Federal regulations and very few Federal enforcement actions under FDCA Section 403(d) are evidence that Section 403(d) is not being adequately implemented by FDA. In fact, these groups believe that, taken together, this lack of FDA action is yet another example of the "federal government's failure to implement the law adequately" (CSPI/CNI/CFA/NCL, 1991).

One consumer group, the Center for Science in the Public Interest (CSPI) stated that

> the language of the [FDCA] lacks specific guidance as to what constitutes a misleading container, making it extremely difficult to prosecute violations without adequate regulations. In fact, the FDA has not initiated a case under this section of the [FDCA] in over 30 years (the last case initiated under Section 403(d) was brought in 1958) (Lindan, 1991, p. 3).

Further, CSPI and other consumer groups support legislative initiatives, similar to that proposed by New York, to prevent downsizing of packages by food manufacturers (CSPI/CNI/CFA/NCL, 1991).

Conclusions

The deliberations of the Committee regarding FDCA Section 403(d) were among its most extensive. The Committee found that notwithstanding FDA's decision to rely solely on the statutory provision of Section 403(d) and generally ignored the section, only a few States have taken independent action to establish their own requirements for slack fill and deceptive packaging. Yet, at the same time, a wide divergence of views exists among State officials, industry, and consumer groups regarding the adequacy of FDA's regulatory program. Consumer groups believe strongly that this provision of the law is not being adequately implemented whereas industry groups strongly believe that implementation of this Section is adequate. State officials provided the Committee with several examples of packages of food products that are currently being marketed, and represent, in their view, objectionable packaging practices that have occurred under FDA's current policies.

The Committee was impressed by the examples of packaging provided by State officials; such examples also lent support to the strong positions taken by consumer groups. The Committee recognized that FDA's lack of success in bringing actions (FDA has lost all court cases pertaining to slack fill) may have influenced the agency's efforts in this area. Moreover, relatively few States have established more specific requirements related to slack fill and deceptive packaging, suggesting a satisfaction on their part with Federal requirements as established by Section 403(d).

Ultimately, two divergent views emerged within the Committee as well. One view was that, in the absence of evidence of a meaningful level of consumer deception, it is inappropriate to suggest that FDA expend limited resources to issue regulations to solve a problem that can be addressed adequately under present law. The examples of deceptive packaging presented to the Committee that had the most vivid impact could have been addressed quite readily under current law. Since the Committee concluded that enforcement would not be examined as an element of adequacy, new regulations should not be suggested on the basis of FDA's decision not to enforce present law more aggressively.

The alternative view was that deceptive or slack filled containers are to be considered a matter of national importance and the perception on the part of State officials and consumer groups that there is a problem supports that conclusion. It was the position of some Committee members that FDA might have been more successful in subsequent litigation had its policies and expectations of industry been adequately enunciated following the loss of the cases noted above. The matter was finally resolved by expressing the majority view of the Committee; the results are apparent in the following conclusions.

Based on its analysis and criteria, the Committee concludes that FDA implementation of FDCA Section 403(d) has not been adequate and that no single State's requirement is adequate for adoption as a Federal requirement. Given the California experience as an example, the Committee would argue that FPLA language provides FDA with a means to implement the intent of FDCA Section 403(d). Therefore, the Committee suggests that FDA consider using the FPLA definition for nonfunctional slack fill as a guide for interpreting and enforcing FDCA Section 403(d). The Committee further concluded that State requirements related to FDCA Section 403(d) be exempted from preemption until a formal FDA policy is in place.

PLACEMENT OF REQUIRED INFORMATION—SECTION 403(f)

FDCA Section 403(f) states that a food is misbranded

if any word, statement, or other information required by or under authority of this act to appear on the label or labeling is not prominently placed thereon with such conspicuousness and in such terms as to render it likely to be read and understood by the ordinary individual under customary conditions of purchase and use.

Federal Requirements

FDA's regulations implementing FDCA Section 403(f) are found at 21 CFR Part 101. Specific regulations include the placement of mandatory information (e.g., product name, net weight, ingredients, name and address of manufacturer, etc.) and specifications for type size.

Section 101.1 — Principal Display Panel

The principal display panel "shall be large enough to accommodate all the mandatory label information required . . . with clarity and conspicuousness and without obscuring design, vignettes, or crowding." This section also defines the location and size requirements for the PDP. A minimum type size of 1/16 inch is required for all information appearing on the principal display panel.

Section 101.2 — Information Panel

The information panel shall be "immediately contiguous and to the right of the principal display panel." A minimum type size of 1/16 inch is required for all information appearing on the information panel.

Section 101.3 — Identity Labeling of Food

The "statement of the identity of the commodity" shall be a primary feature on the principal display panel. This section defines prominence of the statement size and location on the panel.

Case Law

The Committee found only three Federal court cases that interpret FDCA Section 403(f). In *U.S. v. 46 Cases,* 204 F.Supp 321, 323 (D.R.I.1962), the court held that a manufacturer would be in compliance with FDCA Section 403(f)

> in a particular case if [its label] statements are prominent enough to be seen and understood by the ordinary individual who is interested in discovering and learning the information disclosed thereby, and who makes a minimum examination of the package to determine its net weight and the ingredients of the [food] contained in said package.

The required statements in this case were printed on the label in a distinctive color that was not used for any other statements appearing on the package, and easily readable at a distance of approximately 29 inches by an average person. The manufacturer thus met the requirements of Section 403(f).

In contrast, when required information cannot be read without the aid of a magnifying glass, *U.S. v. 70 Gross Bottles,* Civ. No. 2365 (S.D.Ohio 1952), or it is printed in such small type on such a background as to be practically invisible, *U.S. v. 274 Boxes,* No. 14769 (D.N.J.1950), the food is considered misbranded under FDCA Section 403(f).

State Requirements

At least 34 States have misbranding regulations that pertain to prominence, and the Committee identified a total of 96 State regulations and 2 pending bills. The great majority (78.1 percent) of State prominence regulations are targeted to specific foods, such as oleomargarine, and require that a product prominently and conspicuously place required information on the label. Most often, the required information specifies the exact nomenclature, such as "oleomargarine" or "ice milk," to be placed on a product's label. Required type size and font are often specified in State regulations.

Dairy Products—Substitutes

Dairy product substitutes account for the largest group (a total of 48) of State regulations establishing prominence requirements. These regulations primarily establish specific product nomenclature that must appear on the product's label following specific criteria.

Eighteen States have regulations on oleomargarine/margarine.[1] Many States require a minimum type size, and some even require a specific type font. In Indiana, for example, the name must be in plain Gothic letters of

---

[1] Ark. Stat. Ann. §20-59-201, §20-59-306; Cal. Food & Agric. Code §39471, §39501, §39521, §39382, §39411, §39432; Colo. Rev. Stat. §35-24-115; Conn. Gen. Stat. §21a-16; Del. Code Ann. Title 16, §3310; Iowa Code §191.2; Idaho Code §37-328, §37-331 to 37-332b, §37-333; Ind. Code §16-1-34-3; Kan. Stat. Ann. §65-639; Mass. Gen. Stat. Ann. §49; Mich. Comp. Laws §12.742; Minn. Stat. §33.06; Miss. Code Ann. §75-31-21; Nev. Rev. Stat. §584.165, §584.170, §584.175; N.Y. Agric. & Mkts. Law §62; Pa. Cons. Stat. Ann. Title 31, §800-4b; Vt. Stat. Ann. Title 6, §3441 and 3442; Wis. Stat. §97.18.

a type size not less than 20 points. An additional 12 State regulations focus on renovated or substitute butter, most often specifying type size and font.[2]

In Mississippi, as an example, renovated butter must be marked as such in plain Gothic letters at least 3/8 inch high on two sides of each container (Miss. Code Ann. §75-31-17, §75-31-423). Alabama requires substitutes for butter to declare "substitute for butter" in black Gothic letters not less than 1 inch high and 1 inch wide (Ala. Code §2-13-17). There are 18 other State regulations that establish labeling requirements for reduced fat cheeses, ice milk, skim milk, nondairy products, or products in semblance of frozen desserts.[3]

Blended Products

Twenty State regulations have been issued pertaining to the nomenclature and labeling of blends or mixtures. Seven States have prominence regulations for honey products.[4] Three States regulate oils that are mixtures or blends (Cal. Food & Agric. Code §28475 to 28478, §28480 to 28482, §28484 to 28486; Mass. Gen. Stat. Ann. §61; 7 Pa. Code §47.2 and 47.3). For example, California's olive oil regulation has specific requirements on the declaration required for any olive oil blended with other edible oils. Three States have prominence regulations on blended vinegars (Mass. Ann. Laws Ch. 94, §186 and 187; Minn R. 1550.0640; N.Y. Agric. & Mkts. Law §209).

The six remaining prominence regulations regarding blends or mixtures vary in scope and effect.[5] In Massachusetts, for example, any maple product sold that consists of maple syrup in combination with other ingredients must be labeled with a statement in which all the ingredients appear in the same size type as the words "maple syrup" (Mass. Gen. Stat. Ann. §36C).

---

[2] Ala. Code §2-13-20; Conn. Gen. Stat. §21a-20; Idaho Code §37-328, §37-331 to 37-332b, §37-333; Mass. Gen. Stat. Ann. §59; Miss. Code Ann. §75-31-17, §75-31-423; Mo. Rev. Stat. §196.775; N.H. Rev. Stat. Ann. §184.47; Utah Code Ann. §4-3-14.

[3] Ala. Code §2-13-17; Ark. Stat. Ann. §20-59-235; Ariz. Rev. Stat. Ann. §3-326, §36-906.14; Cal. Food & Agric. Code §39151, §39152, §39181, §39211, §39213; Fla. Stat. §503.011, §503.031, §503.062; Idaho Code §37-326; Minn. Stat. §32.62, §32.481, §32.5311; Minn. R. 1550.0620; N.D. Cent. Code §4-30-41.1 to 4-30-41.3; N.H. Rev. Stat. Ann. §184.52; Or. Rev. Stat. §621-425; Pa. Code §61.65; Vt. Stat. Ann. Title 6, §2811.

[4] Ala. Code §2-13-121, §1-13-122; Conn. Gen. Stat. §22-181a; Mont. Code. Ann. §50-31-204; N.Y. Agric. & Mkts. Law §205 and 206; 31 Pa. Stat. §382; Tex. Agric. Code §131.011, §131.081 to 131.084; Washington Rev. Code §69.28.400.

[5] Iowa Code §189.11; Mass. Gen. Stat. Ann. §36C; Minn. R. 1550.0600; S.D. Cod. Laws Ann. §39-4-15; Vt. Stat. Ann. Title 6, §493; W.Va. Code §16-7-2.

Disclosure of Colors, Flavors, and Preservatives

The Committee identified five States that have issued specific regulations on the prominent disclosure of any artificial colors, flavors, or chemical preservatives in food products.[6] This area duplicates several Federal and State requirements related to FDCA Section 403(k). For example, Pennsylvania requires nonalcoholic beverages with artificial colors, flavors, or sweeteners to be conspicuously labeled as such (31 Pa. Code §790.7), and requires that added color in food be conspicuously declared on labels using such phrases as "artificially colored," "certified color added," "vegetable dye added," or "color added" (7 Pa. Code §43.5).

Other Prominence Regulations

Thirteen other State regulations require the prominent labeling of various kinds of product information.[7] Minnesota, for example, has regulations (Minn. R. 1550.0920) requiring products of substandard quality or below standard of fill to include statements to that effect in a prominent manner that parallels Federal requirements under FDCA Section 403(h) (see the later discussion).

Connecticut and Pennsylvania (Conn. Gen. Stat. §42-115j-6; Pa. Cons. Stat. Ann. Title 31, §4) set forth general requirements for placement and prominence of required information. All information required to appear on a package in Connecticut must be prominent, definite, and plain; the statute also requires that it be conspicuous as to size and style of letters and numbers, and the color of the letters and numbers contrast with the background color. In Pennsylvania, a wide variety of required messages must be located on the main label of each package, in type not smaller than 8-point Brevier capital letters.

---

[6] Ariz. Rev. Stat. Ann. §36-973; Minn. R. 1550.0870; 7 Pa. Code §43.5; 31 Pa. Stat. §790.7; S.D. Cod. Laws Ann. §39-4-5.

[7] Conn. Gen. Stat §42-115j-6; Haw. Rev. Stat. §328-41, §328-47, §328.62; Iowa Code §190.11; Mass. Ann. Laws Ch. 94, §117G; Mass. Gen. Stat. Ann. §154 and §155; Minn. R. 1550. 0920; Minn. Stat. §28.07; N.J. bill no. 4880 (pending); N.Y. Agric. & Mkts. Law §211; N.Y. Senate bill no. 5081 (pending), Assembly no. 7296 (pending); Pa. Cons. Stat. Ann. Title 31, §4; Tex. health & Safety Code Ann. §436.08; Wash. Rev. Code §69.28.100; Wis. Stat. §97.57.

Industry Perspective

Although numerous industry representatives stated their belief that FDA has adequately implemented the six provisions of FDCA Section 403 under study, only the NFPI specifically noted that FDA had more than adequately implemented FDCA Section 403(f). The Institute stated that the agency "has established a regulation expressly governing minimum typesize for product label features. FDA also specifies throughout the regulation where certain information must appear and that information must appear together" (NFPI, 1991).

Consumer Perspective

The Center for Science in the Public Interest (CSPI) stated in a letter to the Committee that "[w]hile [Federal] regulations address many important issues, they are insufficient. . . . [T]he regulations do not address other problems with the format of required label information which make the label difficult to read. For example, the regulations do not address the problems of writing that is in all capital letters or that has a flush right margin" (Lindan, 1991).

Conclusions

In its analysis of this Section, the Committee concluded that FDA's regulations utilize a balance of location, continuity, size, and ink color to establish standard and predictable formats for food labeling.

Based on its analysis and criteria, the Committee believes that most of the State regulations related to FDCA Section 403(f) are designed to protect specific industries (see criterion 4, Chapter 4). Many of the products for which requirements exist are substitutes for products of special economic importance within a State. None appeared to meet a legitimate specific local consumer need, thereby qualifying them as candidates for exemption. As an example (although many of these requirements may now be preempted), some State prominence regulations require the use of pejorative terms (i.e., "imitation" low-fat frozen desserts), which might deter consumers from purchasing the foods. This requirement conflicts with current public health efforts to encourage Americans to purchase and consume lower-fat products. Where not preempted, State requirements of this type should be discouraged by FDA. **Based on its analysis and criteria, the Committee concludes that FDCA Section 403(f) is adequately implemented. The Committee further** concludes that State requirements related to FDCA Section 403(f) are candidates for preemption.

One general principle that FDA should consider adopting relates to the specificity that often characterizes State prominence regulations, including specific requirements for minimum type size, font, and contrasting colors for background versus print of required material. These specifics eliminate ambiguity about possible violations of the prominence regulation and thus simplify compliance. FDA's current regulations do not provide as precise a definition for "conspicuous" and "prominent" as do some States. Therefore, this lack of definition may leave greater latitude for industry to interpret such regulations as broadly as it chooses and could place a greater enforcement burden on FDA. Although FDA should allow manufacturers a reasonable degree of flexibility, the Committee suggests that FDA review the results of recent studies on the readability of product information and consider whether the recommendations provided in these studies offer options to improve consumer use of product information (AARP, 1986; NDMA, 1990, 1991; Eskin, 1991).

STANDARDS OF QUALITY AND OF FILL OF CONTAINER—SECTION 403(h)

FDCA Section 403(h) provides that a food is misbranded

if it purports to be or is represented as—

(1) a food for which a standard of quality has been prescribed by regulations as provided by section 401, and its quality falls below such standard, unless its label bears, in such manner and form as such regulations specify, a statement that it falls below such standard; or

(2) a food for which a standard or standards of fill of container have been prescribed by regulations as provided by section 401, and it falls below the standard of fill of container applicable thereto, unless its label bears, in such manner and form as regulations specify, a statement that it falls below such standard.

Federal Requirements

Section 403(h) must be read in conjunction with FDCA Section 401. Section 401 authorizes FDA to establish by regulation reasonable definitions and standards of identity, standards of quality, and/or standards of fill of container for any food. FDCA Section 403(h) protects consumers by requiring that when foods with established standards of quality and/or fill of container fail to meet those standards, they must be labeled as substandard.

Regulations that provide general statements of substandard quality and fill of container, 21 CFR §130.14, have been promulgated under Section 403(h). Specifications include the exact wording of the required statements:

21 CFR § 130.14(a)   "Below Standard in Quality
                      Good Food—Not High Grade"
21 CFR § 130.14(b)   "Below Standard in Fill."

Also specified are the size of the letters (which is dependent on the weight of the package), type style (Cheltenham Bold condensed capital letters), color of the lettering, and placement of the statements. Label statements must be enclosed within rectangles composed of lines not less than 6 points in width on a strongly contrasting, uniform background and placed where they can be easily seen near the food name or picture.

Labeling requirements for foods that have established quality standards, but no standards of identity, are defined at 21 CFR Part 103. Currently, bottled water is the only such product. These regulations specify criteria for levels of microorganisms and physical factors such as turbidity, color, flavor, and odor as indicative of quality. The regulations also provide specific labeling language for foods with established quality standards that fail to meet the standard. The following are examples of these labeling requirements:

"Below Standard in Quality . . . ,"
1. "Contains Excessive Bacteria"
2. "Excessively Turbid"
3. "Abnormal Color" [21 CFR §103.5(b)].

The rarity with which any of the required statements now appear on labels is commonly attributed to their effectiveness as crepe labeling, which deters the marketing of products that do not meet the standards. Standards of quality and fill are frequently components of the more than 300 standards of identity for various foods (21 CFR §130 through §169.182).

Case Law

Only a few court cases have interpreted Section 403(h) directly. A number of other court cases have cited Section 403(h) to illustrate a contrast with Section 403(g), which imposes requirements on foods for which there are standards of identity. The paucity of interpretive case law suggests that most enforcement that has occurred has not resulted in reported decisions. The court has ruled that informative labeling can prevent violation of

Section 403(h) but not of Section 403(g); see, for example, *U.S. v. 62 Cases*, 183 F.2d. 1014, 1017 (10th Cir. 1950); and *U.S. v. 30 Cases*, 93 F.Supp. 764, 770 (S.D.Iowa 1950) *reversed on other grounds*, 340 U.S. 593 (1951).

State Requirements

A review of State labeling requirements in the area of standards of quality and fill of container raised an important question of interpretation of NLEA for the Committee. NLEA seems clear in regard to preemption of State labeling requirements "of the type" for which Federal standards of identity exist. If NLEA also calls for automatic preemption of State requirements for labeling products for which Federal standards of quality and fill of container exist, the question of whether there are State substandard labeling requirements related to FDCA Section 403(h) becomes moot. Further, it is reasonable to conclude that State substandard labeling requirements for foods that are not covered by FDA standards of fill or quality are also not covered by Section 403(h) and therefore not subject to study. The Committee decided to view its jurisdiction in this area broadly and review all State requirements regarding the labeling of products for which State standards of quality and fill of container have been established.

A number of States have regulations regarding standards of fill of container, but most do not establish labeling requirements for foods that do not meet these standards. For example, three States have set standards of fill of container for raw-shucked or canned oysters. Florida has established a maximum free liquor content (15 percent by volume) for containers of raw-shucked oysters [Fla. Admin. Code §5E-6.010(8)(d)]. In New York, a maximum of 10 percent free liquor (by volume) is allowed in containers of raw-shucked oysters (N.Y. Stat. §17-212). Maryland sets its standard at 5 percent (Md. COMAR 01.15.08.02). Minnesota regulation (Minn. R. 1545.2670) requires drained weight of oysters to be no less that 59 percent.

Industry Perspective

No industry representative spoke directly to the adequacy of implementation of FDCA Section 403(h). However, GMA stated that the interrelationships of standards of identity and quality are complex and often impossible to separate. It pointed out that FDA has not attempted to designate which regulations in 21 CFR Parts 131 through 169 relate to quality and which relate to identity (Section 403(h) and Section 401, respectively). Instead, FDA has stated that most (if not all) of these regulations apply to both the FDCA provisions on quality and identity. In GMA's opinion, violations of food standards are undoubtedly concerned with food quality, except for provisions that relate solely to standard of fill of container. Furthermore, in the specific case of bottled water, it believes that no State may require any additional or different requirements for any such product that are not identical to requirements in 21 CFR §103.35 (GMA, 1991).

Consumer Perspective

No consumer group spoke directly to the adequacy of implementation of FDCA Section 403(h) but acknowledged that additional quality standards can be found interspersed with standards of identity and requirements for nonstandardized foods, although these standards only govern specific products. Further, they noted a similar situation for standards of fill. The only general Federal regulations relating to standards of fill pertain to the methodology for measuring the water capacity of containers and a statement of substandard fill. There may also be an occasional reference to a standard of fill interspersed with the regulations for standards of identity and common or usual name (CSPI/CNI/CFA/NCL, 1991).

Conclusions

FDA has regulations that establish adequate procedures for labeling products that fail to meet standards of quality and fill of container. Rarely are products found that contain the required statements set forth under FDCA Section 403(h), because of both the imparted inferior connotation of a product with "crepe labeling" and the link between standards of identity and fill for many products. **Based on its analysis and criteria, the Committee concludes that FDCA Section 403(h) is adequately implemented. The Committee further concludes that State requirements related to FDCA Section 403(h) are candidates for preemption.**

Because of the ambiguities of NLEA regarding preemption of State standards of quality and of fill of container requirements for labeling "of the type," FDA should consult with Congress to clarify their status for the States and industry.

COMMON OR USUAL NAME—SECTION 403(i)(1)

FDCA Section 403(i)(1) states that a food is misbranded "if it is not subject to the provisions of paragraph (g) of this section [which concerns standards of identity] unless its label bears (1) the common or usual name, if any there be."

A similar requirement is found in FPLA Section 4(a)(1), which specifies that each consumer commodity—packaged food, in this context—must "bear a label specifying the identity" of the product. The "common or usual name" required under FDCA constitutes the statement of identity required under FPLA [Sections 4(a)(1) and 5(c)(3)].

Federal Requirements

For more than 50 years, the regulation of food nomenclature has been a difficult and contentious issue for manufacturers and regulators (and the Committee found it no less so in its own deliberations). FDCA authorized the development of "standards of identity" that, in effect, are legally mandated recipes that standardize the composition and names of common products. Standards of identity were established for a large number of foods following passage of the 1938 Act. By the early 1950s, nearly half of foods purchased were "standardized" foods (i.e., those for which a standard of identity had been established; Lorman, 1990). Because of the cumbersome administrative process for creating and modifying standards of identity, however, in the mid-1970s, FDA began to address issues of nomenclature regulation primarily through the use of formalized "common or usual names" (Hutt and Merrill, 1991).

Thus, FDA has published a definition of common or usual names and provided a mechanism by which such a name for a food can be established by regulation. Section 403(i)(1) is implemented mainly through regulations at 21 CFR §101.3, which deal with the identity of packaged food, and 21 CFR Part 102, which provide principles for the designation of common or usual names and contain the names of foods for which they have been established by regulation (Table 5-1). The general principles behind the use and development of common or usual names are delineated at 21 CFR §102.5. CFR §101.3(b)(3) specifies that a packaged food shall bear, in the absence of a common or usual name, "an appropriately descriptive term, or when the nature of the food is obvious, a fanciful name commonly used by the public for such food." FDA essentially stopped adopting common or usual names for foods in the late 1970s.

TABLE 5-1 Foods Listed in 21 CFR Part 102, Common or Usual Names for
Nonstandardized Foods

Food Item	CFR Section
Peanut spreads	102.23
Frozen "heat and serve" dinners	102.26
Foods packaged for use in the preparation of "main dishes" or "dinners"	102.28
Noncarbonated beverage products containing no fruit or vegetable juices	102.30
Diluted orange juice	102.32
Diluted fruit or vegetable juice beverages other than diluted orange juice	102.33
Mixtures of edible fat or oil and olive oil	102.37
Onion rings made from diced onions	102.39
Potato chips made from dried potatoes	102.41
Fish sticks or portions made from minced fish	102.45
Pacific whiting	102.46
Fried clams made from minced clams	102.49
Crabmeat	102.50
Seafood cocktail	102.54
Nonstandardized breaded composite shrimp units	102.55
Greenland turbot	102.57

NOTE: CFR = Code of Federal Regulations.

Petitions Regarding Common or Usual Names

As outlined in 21 CFR Part 102.19, FDA may issue, amend, or revoke
regulations prescribing a common or usual name for a food. Any persons,
such as manufacturers or State/local governments, may petition FDA to
establish a common or usual name for new or substitute foods, as discussed
below. Regardless of the extent of preemption of State/local laws and
regulations, NLEA does not impair the ability of manufacturers or
State/local governments to petition FDA for issuance or modification of a
common or usual name.

FDA provided the Committee with examples of manufacturers' petitions
and agency decisions with respect to establishing common or usual names.
Denials of petitions by FDA have frequently been based on the potential for
economic deception of consumers, if use of the requested common or usual
name were to be allowed. Perhaps the most notable characteristic of these
documents, however, is the rate at which the petitions were processed.
Although FDA regulations ostensibly require a response in 180 days, and
some were processed even faster, more than 6 and up to 24 months

frequently elapsed before a decision was issued. The limited data reviewed by the Committee also seem to show that petitions are denied more frequently by FDA than they are adopted.

Imitation, Alternative, and Substitute Food Products

Since passage of the 1938 Act, any food product that was similar to but did not meet a standard of identity was required by FDCA Section 403(c) to be termed "imitation," regardless of the relative food values of the standard and nonstandard product. Because the term "imitation" was generally viewed by consumers as negative and perceived as inferior, many substitute products that might have been marketed were abandoned by food manufacturers. Following recommendations made at the 1969 White House Conference on Food, Nutrition, and Health during revision of FDA's labeling policies in the early 1970s, a change in emphasis occurred, and the word *imitation* was required only to reflect nutritional inferiority of the substitute product (FDA, 1973b). The agency reaffirmed its position a decade later, rejecting alternative approaches (FDA, 1983). FDA's purpose in using "imitation" in this way was to provide a means by which new products could be given an appropriate descriptive name rather than bearing the demeaning term "imitation" (Hutt, 1989). By the early 1980s, however, FDA was imposing descriptors such as "alternative" and "substitute" on the labeling for products that simulated standardized foods and were nutritionally equivalent but did not meet the standard. This change was a significant departure from the policies adopted in the early 1970s, immediately following the definition of "imitation" to mean nutritional inferiority. Hutt and Merrill offer an interpretation of this change in FDA's policy:

> In the early 1970s, FDA made the decision to apply the same policy on common or usual names to standardized and nonstandardized foods. Previously the agency had taken the position that any new substitute for a standardized food was required to be labeled as an imitation but a new substitute for a nonstandardized food was not required to be so labeled. Under its new policy FDA took the position that the common or usual name for a nonstandardized food could *include* the name of a standardized food, as long as the difference between the products was made clear. This new policy was intended to prevent standards of identity from operating as barriers to the development of new food products, especially new versions of traditional foods with macronutrient composition modified to meet national nutrition goals. Food producers responded by developing dozens of new products with a reduced content of calories, sodium, cholesterol, and fat.
>
> A decade later, however, FDA reverted to the pre-1970 approach. Modified versions of standardized foods were required to be designated as "alternative" or "substitute" products. If a modified product had its own standard of identity, however, the "alternative" or "substitute" language could be omitted. In substance, the agency

substituted the terms "alternative" or "substitute" for the older "imitation" as a way of differentiating between standardized and nonstandardized versions of the same product (Hutt and Merrill, 1991, pp. 156–157).

Although the agency may not agree entirely with the position quoted above, FDA leadership has recognized the possibility that consumers may be misled and confused as a result of the labeling policies of the past 20 years. However, as FDA Commissioner David Kessler recently commented, "There must be an incentive for industry to develop new food products" (Van Wagner, 1991).

State Requirements

Many State statutes or regulations establish or have bearing on the common or usual names of foods, as revealed by the materials provided to the Committee. The discussion below illustrates State requirements currently in effect and outlines the concerns expressed by States regarding FDA implementation.

A number of State agencies expressed concern about the responsiveness of FDA in addressing local nomenclature problems. Many regulators feared that even with the petition process, their ability to deal with certain regulatory problems might be diminished following preemption. One key issue is the overlap among standards of quality, standards of identity, and common or usual names.

In this regard, the Arizona Department of Health Services specifically cited its rule for labeling of bottled water, which is more restrictive than Federal regulations (Ariz. Rev. Stat. Ann. §9R-8-204). The State has rules providing that defined common names be used for bottled water products in addition to quality standards and prefers that these requirements not be preempted (Englender, 1991).

The California Department of Health Services stated that its Health & Safety Code (§26594) establishes definitions and standards for bottled water products that have no similar Federal definitions. In addition, the California Code of Regulations (§15825) provides that shrimp, crab, and seafood cocktails must have at least 30 percent of the defining item and a pH of 3.70 (Sheneman, 1991).

The Connecticut Department of Consumer Protection reported several areas of common or usual name regulation that were of concern relative to preemption, including (1) names for certain meats (Conn. St. Regs. §21a-102-1 to §21a-102-6), (2) definitions for bottled water products (Conn. St. Regs. §21a-150a to §21a-150j), and (3) labeling of juices and ciders (Conn. St. Regs. §21a-146 to §21a-148). Connecticut recommended that FDA adopt standards either equal to or more stringent than those currently in effect in the State (Schaffer, 1991).

Florida's Department of Agriculture and Consumer Services (FDACS) stated that:

> There is a great deal of abuse in the market place with respect to common or usual name declaration. . . . Frequently rather than develop a fanciful name or unique identifier for a new food, the food is identified in relation to a standardized or commonly recognized food. Examples are designer foods which are formulated to meet a specific health issue and diluted juice beverages or fruit flavored beverages . . . the regulations with respect to common or usual names are inadequate and currently provide for consumer confusion, misrepresentation and fraud" (Crawford, 1991).

FDACS identified several areas in which preemption could occur and questions might be raised about the level of protection offered by the Federal statutes: whether (1) regulations for unenriched bakery, cereal grain, and pasta products would be permitted; (2) the quality standards of Florida's Bottled Water Law would be enforceable (the law provides both standards of identity and quality that exceed Federal standards); and (3) FDA through its rulemaking process would follow the FDACS recommendation to adopt portions of the Florida Citrus Code to provide what Florida views as greater consumer protection than Federal statutes (Crawford, 1991; FDACS, 1991).

The Georgia Department of Agriculture (GDA) considered FDCA and its implementing regulations generally adequate but expressed concern that "there is no enforcement being taken in this area" (Niles, 1991a). It provided examples that included the marketing of "soybean cheese products" that are specifically excluded under Federal standards of identity and the failure of FDA to address deception in the area of bottled water. GDA argued further that

> the common or usual name of the food has become unenforceable; dairy products with standards of identity are being manipulated and no longer meet standards of identity, nonstandardized foods are out of control, and in many cases, are meaningless. This is an area which seems impossible to regulate, and is creating chaos in the food business (Niles, 1991a).

Thus, adequacy and uniformity of enforcement at the Federal level seem to be the key to the acceptance of preemption on the part of the States with respect to common or usual names. In another communication, GDA discussed issues and concerns regarding the labeling of bottled water (Niles, 1991b). Ray Niles, Assistant Director of GDA, indicated that the issues with respect to the labeling of spring versus well water were mainly economic and did not pertain to public health. He indicated that Georgia, along with other

States, would not be in favor of preemption of its regulations regarding the labeling of spring water.

As an expression of concern over preemption, the Hawaii Department of Health has submitted a request for exemption of its standards pertaining to bottled water, milk, poi, oriental noodles, and frozen desserts (Tamura, 1991). Each of these matters pertains to food standards and, potentially, common or usual names.

The Maine Department of Agriculture reported two areas of its regulations that concern nomenclature (Davis, 1991). Its cider labeling law would be preempted unless a waiver is requested. In addition, Maine's common or usual names for surimi products would be preempted.

The Michigan Department of Agriculture indicated that FDCA is "adequate in concept although [it] lacks clarity" with respect to several areas including common or usual names (Heffron, 1991). The agency indicated that labeling of diluted fruit beverages is an example of lack of uniformity "that could easily be from vagueness in requirements (and also from a lack of enforcement efforts of any kind)." As Frank (1991) suggests, conflicts exist between Michigan's Regulation No. 549, which defines a variety of juice-based beverages, and the common or usual names proposed by FDA.

The Nevada Department of Human Resources Health Division stated that the impact of preemption would be minimal in that State because it considers the Federal statutes adequate (Nebe, 1991).

The South Dakota Department of Health and Department of Commerce and Regulation reported that existing State food and beverage statutes would be preempted. These agencies felt that Federal food and beverage requirements would be more stringent than those currently in effect and thus would provide better protection (Senger, 1991).

The Utah Department of Agriculture identified problems related to deceptive brand names, trade names, and trademarks. The Department argued that these issues provide an "opportunity for consumer confusion" (McClellan, 1991). The Vermont Department of Agriculture stated concerns related mainly to the naming of maple syrup products (Dunsmore, 1991).

Appendix H provides additional information on selected commodities and details about State/local versus Federal common or usual name requirements.

Industry Perspective

Representatives of the food industry have indicated that "the regulations in Section 101.3 and Part 102 (of the CFR) provide an entirely adequate federal system for regulating common or usual names," with the exception of cases that involve modification of standardized foods (GMA, 1991). GMA also stated that "any state requirement relating to a common or usual name for a food product that is not identical with the Federal requirement [will] be preempted [by NLEA]."

A similar opinion was voiced by Kraft General Foods; that is, after the date of preemption under NLEA,

> if a state considers it necessary to create a regulation which parallels or is identical to the FDA's section 102.5 governing common or usual names (or any other FDA regulation applicable to statements of identity), that State regulation will be required to specify that such product names may be established either through common usage by industry, or through resort to a Federal regulation as prescribed by section 102.5(d). We submit that there can be no other interpretation of the section 6 admonition that no state may *directly or indirectly* establish or continue in effect any type of product name requirement that is not *identical* to the FDA's requirement (KGF, 1991).

Consumer Perspective

Consumer groups have raised a number of issues regarding the adequacy of FDA's common or usual name provisions. In a joint statement to the Committee, four consumer groups indicated that

> improperly identifying food poses a health hazard to consumers with allergies, high cholesterol or other health conditions for which accurate identification of the product is essential. In addition, improper implementation of these sections [of FDCA labeling provisions] permits economic deception by allowing companies to misname inferior, less expensive products in the hope that they will be mistaken for those of higher quality (CSPI/CNI/CFA/NCL, 1991).

With respect to common or usual names, consumer groups have pointed out that regulations are sporadic and insufficient to address all concerns in this area. As shown in Table 5-1, there are only 17 regulations for nonstandardized foods (in 21 CFR Part 102), eight of which deal with fish and seafood (CSPI/CNI/CFA/NCL, 1991).

In contrast, the Arizona Consumers Council (Rudd, 1991) indicated that Federal regulation of common or usual names appeared adequate.

General Conclusions

Based on its analysis and criteria, the Committee concludes that an adequate procedure currently exists in 21 CFR Part 102 for the development and application of common or usual names under FDCA Section 403(i)(1).

The Committee further concludes that State requirements for the process of establishing and defining a common or usual name are candidates for preemption. However, to promote the development and introduction of new foods, the Committee suggests that FDA should more aggressively pursue regulatory options that will allow the formal naming of new, nonstandardized foods.

Discussion of Common and Usual Names for Specific Foods

Having reached the general conclusions detailed above, the Committee discussed whether it had an obligation to review and comment on State requirements for specific foods. Here, as in its discussions of FDCA Section 403(d), the Committee failed to reach unanimity. One position put forth was that although it would be appropriate to examine specific foods to determine whether FDA is adequately implementing FDCA Section 403(i)(1), the conclusion that adequate implementation has occurred should then end the inquiry. Further, the Committee, having concluded that the general principles concerning common or usual names serve to adequately implement the statutory goal of Section 403(i)(1), suggests that it will be FDA's prerogative, under NLEA, to conclude whether all State common or usual name requirements are preempted. These members also felt that a discussion of specific State food requirements by the Committee would only serve to cause confusion because after first concluding that FDA had adequately implemented Section 403(i)(1), the Committee would then specify ways in which it allegedly had not.

The issue as to whether the Committee would continue its study of Section 403(i)(1) by including State requirements for specific foods was a matter of considerable debate. The majority of the Committee concluded that it should view its jurisdiction broadly and review State requirements that establish specific names for foods. The Committee conceded that the results of such a review might further exacerbate concerns expressed over the differences between standards of identity and common or usual names. However, because of the frequency with which these foods were mentioned by States, industry, and consumer groups as having requirements that differed from Federal standards (if any exist), the Committee elected to summarize these issues in the following discussion and provide suggestions to FDA based on its review.

The Committee selected the following food categories for review related to State requirements for common or usual names because of their economic or public health importance, prominence by virtue of the number of State requirements that address them, regional significance, or fulfillment in some other fashion of the criteria established by the Committee.

Bottled Water

The regulation of bottled water requires consideration of two provisions of FDCA that Congress has directed should be studied: the requirement that a food not subject to a standard of identity bear a common or usual name (if any there be) [FDCA Section 403(i)(1)], and the requirement that a food meet any applicable standard of quality or disclose on its label that it does not [FDCA Section 403(h)(1)]. This discussion examines whether FDA has adequately implemented the statutory provisions of FDCA Section 403(i)(1) (for additional information on bottled water requirements, see Appendix I).

In 1973, FDA exercised its authority under FDCA Section 401 and established quality standards for bottled water. In proposing the standards, FDA explained that "bottled water is increasingly being used as a source of drinking water. . . . The consumer expects bottled water to meet the minimum criteria established for public drinking water supplies" (FDA, 1973a). The agency based the quality standards on the 1962 Public Health Service standards for public drinking water supplies. It noted that the recently created Environmental Protection Agency (EPA) had assumed the responsibility for establishing drinking water standards and FDA intended to revise the bottled water standards to keep them compatible with the EPA standards.

When FDA first proposed a standard of quality for bottled water, the agency departed from its usual procedures of proposing a standard of identity at the same time. (The bottled water quality standard is the only quality standard FDA ever adopted without at the same time adopting a standard of identity.) The agency's initial *Federal Register* notice did not explain its rationale for this decision, but several commentors urged FDA to regulate the use of identifying terms such as "spring," "well," and "distilled water." FDA declined, stating that

there is no need for a requirement that the source of treatment of the water be declared on the label of bottled water. Bottled drinking water can be produced from various sources of water, and various types of treatment of the water can be used in manufacturing bottled water of an acceptable quality. If the manufacturer decides to provide information in the labeling or in advertising relating to bottled water, stating or implying that it is the product of a specific source of water or that the water has been treated in a specific manner, such information must be truthful, factual, and not misleading in any respect. Section 403(a) of the act provides that a food shall be deemed to be misbranded if its labeling is false or misleading in any particular. The Commissioner concludes that this statutory authority is sufficient to provide for

regulatory action in instances where false or misleading statements concerning the
source or treatment of bottled water are made and that specific statements to this
effect in the standard are unnecessary (FDA, 1973a, p. 32561).

Although several parties filed objections to the final rule, FDA concluded
that they did not justify changing the regulation or conducting a hearing, and
the quality standard became effective on June 19, 1975 (FDA, 1975).

In 1974, passage of the Safe Drinking Water Act codified the division
of labor between FDA and EPA for regulating water. In addition to
directing EPA to promulgate National Primary Drinking Water Standards,
the Safe Drinking Water Act also added Section 410 to FDCA. Section 410
directs FDA to consult with EPA whenever the latter issues interim or
revised national primary drinking water standards and, within 180 days of
EPA's promulgations, to either amend the bottled water standard or explain
in the *Federal Register* why it was not doing so. In 1975, FDA adopted Good
Manufacturing Practice (GMP) regulations for bottled water, including
bottled mineral water (21 CFR §129.1 *et seq.*). Among other things, these
regulations specify the kinds of facilities that must be used and process
controls that are required to ensure a safe product. Recently, as part of
hearings before the House Committee on Energy and Commerce's
Subcommittee on Oversight and Investigations, FDA indicated that it was
reconsidering the coverage of the bottled water standards to include mineral
water and the water component in flavored beverage products fabricated
from bottled water ingredients. The agency further noted that it was
considering a new quality standard to require the water component of such
products as seltzer, tonic water, and colas to meet quality standards based
on EPA's primary drinking water standards (Shank, 1991).

A total of 16 States have expressed their dissatisfaction with FDA's
regulation of bottled water by adopting laws or regulations to provide
additional controls. These laws vary, but in general they address two basic
issues: the nomenclature of various types of bottled waters and the purity
of these products.[8] Many States have adopted the model bottled water
regulation of the Association of Food and Drug Officials (AFDO) or some
variation of it. This regulation contains definitions for artesian well, bottled,
demineralized, drinking, light mineral, mineral, mineralized, natural, purified,
spring, and well water. It requires that all bottled waters bear one of the

---

[8] Ariz. Ag. Rule 290.063 R9-8-204; Cal. Health & Safety Code §26591 to §26594; Conn.
Gen. Stat. Ann. §21a-150; Del. Code Ann. §4315; Fla. Admin. Rule 500.455; Haw. Rev. Stat.
§328D-6; La. Rev. Stat. Ann.§608(12) and reg. 49:2.1110; Me. Rev. Stat. Ann. Title 36, §1572;
Md. Code Ann. §21-336; Miss. reg. §15.18; Mont. Code Ann. §50-31-236; N.J. Stat. Ann. §24:12-
9; N.D. Cent. Code §19-08-02; Ohio Rev. Code Ann. Title 9, §913.24; Okla. Stat. Ann. §1-917;
Tex. Rule §229.81 to §229.88.

defined names and that artificially carbonated waters disclose the addition of carbonation. The model rule also requires compliance with the FDA standard of quality and the bottled water GMPs. In addition, it requires source water and finished product sampling (AFDO, 1984).

In communications to the Committee, a number of States and representatives of consumer groups expressed discontent with FDA's inaction in the face of false and misleading labeling claims for bottled water products. Further, the Committee found that even a cursory examination of supermarket shelves confirmed that a number of products might be the subject of FDA enforcement action. Much of the concern being expressed stems from the recent growth of the bottled water industry, which has made the public and regulators more aware of potentially false and misleading labeling for bottled water products (Prakash, 1991; Weisenberger, 1991).

Conclusions FDA's original decision not to define the various kinds of bottled water may have been correct when it was adopted in 1973, but the market for, and the public perception of, bottled water have changed substantially since then. The proliferation of products in the marketplace and the increasingly aggressive claims made for those products have magnified the opportunity for public confusion, indicating that the existing policy is not adequate. **Therefore, the Committee suggests that FDA establish common or usual names or standards of identity for bottled water and concludes that State laws and regulations that define and/or standardize the names of the various kinds of bottled water be considered candidates for preemption *after* a Federal requirement is established. The Committee further suggests that AFDO's model bill be examined as a unifying basis for Federal regulation of bottled water.**

Cider, Cider Vinegar, and Other Vinegar Products

A number of States have established requirements for cider, cider vinegar, and other vinegar products. These requirements fall generally into several categories: definitions of the quality and type of raw materials allowed in the production of apple cider products, standards for method of processing and acetic acid concentration for vinegar, the methods of heat treatment of cider, and common or usual names for cider.

The Committee identified 11 States that regulate cider and vinegar products.[9] Maine prohibits the labeling of a product as "cider" if it has been heated at 155°F or higher during production (Me. Rev. Stat. Ann. Title 7, §543-A), and it anticipates preemption unless it petitions for exemption (Davis, 1991). Michigan defines, sets compositional standards and processing and labeling standards for vinegars (Mich. Comp. Laws §289.552 to §289.558).

Conclusions In applying its criteria, the Committee concluded that none of the State requirements it had identified met the threshold for consideration for adoption as a Federal requirement, nor did there appear to be a compelling reason for additional Federal regulation. **Therefore, the Committee concludes that State requirements for cider products are candidates for preemption.**

Citrus Products

There are four primary citrus-producing States (Arizona, California, Florida, and Texas). Florida produces approximately 90 percent of all juice products marketed in the United States. The Florida Department of Agriculture and Consumer Services (FDACS) and the Department of Citrus (FDC) provided the Committee with an extensive analysis of the impact they perceived from the application of NLEA national uniformity provisions to the Florida Citrus Code (FDACS/FDC, 1991). Their analysis identified the central difference between Federal and State regulations to be in grading (not subject of this study) and standards of identity (preempted upon enactment). The responses of the remaining States did not indicate any provisions above and beyond standard labeling requirements or grading standards similar to those of the U.S. Department of Agriculture (USDA).

Conclusions After reviewing Florida's analysis and its current requirements and the provisions of the remaining three citrus-producing States, the Committee concludes that the issues raised by this review fall outside its charge and the State requirements are either already preempted (juice standards of identity) or would not be affected by preemption (grading). The

---

[9] Conn. Gen. Stat. §21a-146 to §21a-148; Iowa Code §190.8, §191.8; Me. Rev. Stat. Ann. §543-A; Mass. Gen. Stat. Ann. §170 and §171; Mich. Comp. Laws §289.552 to §289.558; N.H. Rev. Stat. Ann. §146:14; N.Y. Agric. & Mkts. Law §207 and §208; Ohio Rev. Code Ann. §3715.28 to §3715.33; Pa. Code §921 to §924; R.I. Gen. Laws §21-22-1 to §21-22-3; W.Va. Code §19-22-1, §19-22-5 and §19-22-6.

Committee, however, found merit in Florida's position that its standards of identity may provide additional consumer protection (i.e., specific production criteria beyond FDA's standard of good manufacturing practice). **Therefore, the Committee suggests that Florida and/or other citrus-producing States consider petitioning FDA to amend the Federal standards of identity for citrus products, and existing State requirements be exempt from preemption until the petition process is complete.**

Honey

With the exception of dairy products, more States have regulations for honey than for any other single food.[10] A review of these requirements reveals that a number of States have established grade standards similar to those established by USDA (7 CFR Part 52), microbiological standards, and adulteration regulations. However, most appear to provide economic protection for local industry.

Conclusions Notwithstanding the above evaluation of State requirements for honey, the fact that 23 States decided to specifically regulate this food suggested to the Committee the potential benefit of some Federal unifying regulatory requirement. The promulgation of a Federal standard of identity and quality under FDCA Section 401 would establish national uniformity through clear preemptive action. If appropriate, concerns over the possible microbiological contamination of honey, especially with *Botulinum* spores, might be addressed in a standard of quality established not only under the misbranding provisions but also under the adulteration provisions of FDCA. Such an initiative, however, is not viewed as a high priority among the numerous activities associated with implementation of NLEA. State requirements that establish grades or define adulteration are not subject to study.

---

[10] Ala. Code §2-11-121 and §2-11-122; Ark. Stat. Ann. §20-57-402; Cal. Food & Agric. Code §29401 to §29421, §29448, §29471 to §29474, §29501 to §29504, §29531, §29581 to §29587, §29611 to §29620, §29641 to §29644, §29671 to §29675, §29677; Col. Rev. Stat. §35-25-102 and §35-25-109; Conn. Gen. Stat. §22-181a; Fla. Stat. §582.02, §586.03, §586.051; Ga. Code Ann. §26-2-233; Iowa Code §190.1 and §198.14; Kan. Stat. Ann. §65-681; La. Rev. Stat. §608.1; Minn. Stat. §31.74; Miss. Code Ann. §75-29-601; Nev. Rev. Stat. §583.355; N.H. Rev. Stat. Ann. §429.23; N.M. Stat. Ann. §25-9-263; N.J. Stat. Ann. §205 and §206; N.Y. Agric. & Mktg. Law §206; Ohio Rev. Code Ann. §3715.01, §3715.38; Okla. Stat. Title 78, §81 to 83; Wash. Rev. Code §69.28.020 to 390, §69.28.030, §69.28.400; W.Va. Code §19-20-1 and §19-20-2; Wyo. Stat. §11-8-102.

Therefore, the Committee suggests that FDA consider the need for a single unifying Federal requirement for honey. The Committee further suggests that State requirements for honey be exempted from preemption until a Federal requirement is established.

Milk, Milk Products, and Other Dairy Products

This category of products represented by far the largest number of State requirements. A careful review and evaluation of these requirements, however, led the Committee to the conclusion that all were standards of identity and thus regulated by FDA under FDCA Section 401. **The Committee concludes that the State dairy requirements were preempted upon the date of enactment of NLEA and are not subject to study.** (Appendix G illustrates the abundance of such requirements.)

Seafood

Finfish and Shellfish There are a number of State requirements dealing with common or usual names of seafood (see Appendix H). As noted earlier, of the 17 regulations specified in 21 CFR Part 102 that deal with common or usual names, eight involve seafood (Table 5-1). In an effort to promote uniformity and standardize the confusing and potentially misleading nomenclature of seafood, FDA has issued *The Fish List—FDA Guide to Acceptable Market Names for Food Fish Sold in Interstate Commerce* as a formal advisory opinion (FDA, 1988). This list provides the allowed market name and the scientific and common names for a wide range of common species.[11] Although some criticism has been directed toward the categorization in this list because of the wide range of species within each class, the Committee viewed it as a positive step in providing order in the marketplace.

---

[11] Specific items include capelin/smelt; crabmeat (common or usual name of species defined); kippers; red snapper; lobster, langostino, and crawfish; imitation breaded shrimp; caviar; canned shrimp (size designations); crabmeat products with added fish or other seafood ingredients (e.g., "deviled crabs"); minced fish; Pacific whiting; Greenland turbot and halibut; seafood cocktails; nonstandardized breaded composite shrimp units ("made from minced shrimp" products); fried clams made from minced clams; shellfish, crustaceans, and other aquatic animals (mainly quantity guidelines); imitation crab; processed and/or blended seafood products, including surimi; pollock (cannot be called "snow cod"); Chilean Centolla crab (cannot be called "king crab"); Pacific snapper; golden snapper; tilapia; and calamari/squid.

Particular controversy has developed with respect to nomenclature of red snapper (*Lutjanus campechanus*) owing to the sale of Pacific coast rockfish under the name of red snapper (Otwell, 1985). In response, FDA developed Compliance Policy Guide No. 7108.04, which states:

> BACKGROUND—The name "red snapper" has been preempted by many years of consistent consumer usage as meaning only the fish *Lutjanus campechanus*. Because of the high esteem in which this fish is held by consumers, and the relatively limited catch, there have been numerous attempts to substitute other, less expensive fishes for this species. Substitutes of less desirable species have included members of the family *Lutjanidae*, groupers, a number of West Coast rockfishes of the genus *Sebastes*, and other species. The West Coast rockfishes have, until relatively recently, been distributed mostly locally, and thus have been beyond the reach of the Federal Food, Drug, and Cosmetic Act. Some of the states on the West Coast have officially sanctioned "red snapper" as an alternative name for such members of the *Sebastes* genus, although these fishes are quite different in appearance, flavor, and texture, and are generally regarded by consumers familiar with *Lutjanus campechanus* as inferior.

> POLICY—The labeling or sale of any fish other than *Lutjanus campechanus* as "red snapper" constitutes a misbranding in violation of the Federal Food, Drug, and Cosmetic Act.

Notwithstanding the formal FDA guideline, California still allows the sale of rockfish species under the name of "red snapper" in intrastate commerce.

Several matters of seafood nomenclature have also been addressed by States, which have developed (1) common or usual name regulations for halibut that are identical to the Federal regulations (Alaska Stat. §17.20.045; Mass. Gen. Stat. Ann. §194B; Or. Rev. Stat. §616.217; Wash. Rev. Code §69.04-315); and (2) labeling requirements with respect to the source of catfish (i.e., "farm-raised catfish," "river or lake catfish," "imported catfish," or "ocean catfish") (Ark. Stat. Ann. §20-61-202 and §20-61-206; Miss. Code Ann. §69-7-605 to 69-7-609). FDA's list of acceptable market names further distinguishes between marine species identified as either "ocean catfish" or "sea catfish" (FDA, 1988; NFERF, 1991b). It should be noted that regulatory and promotional aspects of aquaculture per se are under USDA jurisdiction, whereas regulation of harvested catfish and derived food products (including labeling aspects) is handled by FDA.

Surimi-based Imitation Crab and Other Fish Substitutes   Various substitute seafood products pose a labeling problem because of the need to accurately identify products for possible public health reasons (e.g., allergy) and prevent economic deception. With respect to imitation crab products (i.e., products that are defined as not 100 percent crabmeat and often contain surimi manufactured from the processed flesh of pollock or similar fish), such products must be labeled "imitation crabmeat" and bear an appropriately descriptive common or usual name because they are not nutritionally equivalent. In addition, the term "crab legs" has been declared false and misleading when applied to products that contain no crabmeat (NFERF, 1991a).

The NFERF position is based on a guideline issued by FDA with respect to seafood products containing surimi:

POLICY

1. If the surimi-based product purports to be or is represented as a specific type of natural seafood, including shape or form representations, but is nutritionally inferior to that seafood, it must be labeled as imitation. To date FDA has not encountered any surimi-based products in which nutritional equivalency has been achieved.

2. An additional statement of product identity must appear on the principal display panel such as "A blend of fish with _____." The blank is to be filled with the common or usual name of the ingredient or component, such as "snow crab." Because the fish used in the surimi base has been decharacterized, the word "fish" is adequate for the statement of product identity. If an artificial flavor or color is added, the label must so state.

3. The specific names of all seafood used in the product shall appear in the ingredient statement in descending order of predominance ("pollock" must be used as opposed to "white fish"; "snow crab" rather than "crab"). All other ingredients must also be declared in descending order of predominance.

Note: The intermediate surimi product usually contains sugar and/or sorbitol and phosphate compounds as cryoprotectants. These should be listed in the ingredient statement unless removed during the manufacturing process.

4. Products that are not purported or represented to be a specific type of seafood or seafood body part, need not be labeled imitation, but may be marketed if the label properly reflects their composition.

5. Labeling of surimi-based products may suggest use in recipes in place of the natural seafood products by a generalized statement such as, "use like crabmeat, lobster, or shrimp in all seafood recipes," or a similar statement (FDA Compliance Policy Guide No. 7108.16).

Several States have regulations that define various aspects of these issues, including definitions of "crabmeat," and address matters pertaining to "imitation" (Me. Rev. Stat. Ann. Title 12, §6111 and §6112; Md. Health-Gen. Code Ann. §21-340 and §21-341; Tex. Health & Safety Code §436.041, §436.047, §436.048).

Conclusions Nomenclature of seafood is an issue of both public health and economic concern. Identification of species is essential in cases of certain forms of food allergy. In addition, a well-regulated system of common or usual names is essential to prevent economic deception of consumers.

Therefore, the Committee suggests that:

• *The Fish List* **should be continued as a formal FDA advisory opinion to industry.**

- the designations of origin (farm, river, lake) for catfish, which provide potentially useful information to consumers, should be considered by FDA as a candidate for an advisory opinion or incorporated into Federal regulations.
- because FDA policies for labeling surimi-based products appear to provide adequate regulation, State requirements are candidates for preemption.

Miscellaneous State Food Labeling Requirements

The foods listed below are subject to State labeling requirements. Each represents a unique food or a food of special commercial interest and is subject to regulation by only one or two States. They have been grouped in this section for convenience in presenting the Committee's conclusions and recommendations.

Maple Syrup

Two States (N.Y. Agric. & Mkts. Law §203 and §204; Vt. Stat. Ann. Title 6, §481, §492, §493) cited varying requirements related to standards of identity, quality, grading, and common name of origin for maple syrup and related products. In particular, Vermont argued that its standard of identity and grading system for maple syrup and related products were superior to FDA's standard of identity and USDA's grading standards. Both of these issues fall outside of the charge to the Committee.

Conclusions The Committee concludes that the State maple syrup requirements reviewed are either standards of identity and preempted under NLEA Section 6, or grade standards and not subject to NLEA preemption; and therefore, are not subject to study.

Olive and Vegetable Oils

California law requires that products presented as olive oil may be only the oil of the olive tree, in the absence of added color or flavor. The oil may be blended with other oils only if it is clearly labeled (Cal. Health & Safety Code §28475 to §28478, §28480 to §28482, §28454 to §28486). Rhode Island has a similar law that requires identification of blends containing olive oil (R.I. Gen. Laws §21-21-1, §21-21-2, §21-21-6). New York law further requires that oil blends that contain olive oil must be labeled with the percentage of each ingredient (N.Y. Agric. & Mkts. Law §204-a).

Conclusions Federal regulations concerning ingredient labeling and nomenclature of blended oils appear adequate. **Therefore, the Committee concludes that State requirements related to olive oil and oil mixtures are candidates for preemption.**

Oriental Noodles

Hawaiian Administrative Rule §11-29-7 exempts certain oriental noodle products made without egg from Federal standards of identity for macaroni and noodle products (21 CFR Part 139). FDA Compliance Policy Guide 7102.02 (Chow Mein Noodles, Chinese Noodles and Other Oriental Noodles; Labeling), addresses similar issues as the Hawaii rule.

Conclusions Because of national marketing and acceptance of oriental-type noodles, **the Committee suggests that the existing FDA compliance policy guide serve as the national standard for oriental-type noodles and individual State requirements be considered candidates for preemption.**

Pine Nuts

The New Mexico Pinon Nut Act limits the labeling of pinon (or pine) nuts to those from the native pinon tree, *Pinus edulis* and *Pinus monophylla* (N.M. Stat. Ann. §25-10-1 to 3). The Act not only limits labeling to the above species but also provides for a program to promote native pinon nut harvesting and marketing and the future cultivation of local pinon tree varieties.

Conclusions The Committee concludes that although this State provision meets a particular need, it appears to serve only the economic interest of a limited commodity industry. **Therefore, the Committee suggests that New Mexico petition FDA to exempt its pine nut provision from preemption or create a national common or usual name for pinon (pine) nuts.**

Poi

Hawaiian Administrative Rule §11-29-6 defines poi (a paste made from taro root tubers) and provides standards for the percentage of solids in poi and in ready-mixed poi. Hawaii believes that this rule contributes to consumer protection through prevention of economic fraud and adulteration of this unique product.

Conclusions In view of the highly localized and culturally specific nature of poi, **the Committee suggests that Hawaii petition FDA to exempt its poi provision from preemption.**

Vidalia Onions

The State of Georgia has a regulation providing a common or usual name for the Vidalia onion in terms of its botanical identity and locality of production (Ga. Code Ann. §2-14-131 to 2-14-134). Its unique flavor has been credited to the low sulfur soil in the area in which it is grown (Harris, 1983).

Conclusions This State requirement appears to be predominantly protectionist in that no specific justification is provided for limiting the source to the defined producing locality. **However, because of the widespread recognition of the Vidalia onion name, the Committee suggests that Georgia (or any other group or industry) consider submitting a petition to FDA to establish a common or usual name for the Vidalia onion based on measurable geographical, botanical, and/or quality criteria that justifiably differentiate it from other varieties or species of onion.**

Wild Rice

Specific regulations concerning wild rice exist in only two States—Minnesota and Wisconsin (Minn. Stat. §30.49; Wis. Stat. §97.57). These requirements specify the nature of the product and the mode of harvest. Wild rice (botanically a grass) constitutes a minor part of the overall rice market, compared with polished rice, brown rice, and their derived products and is only a minor part of the American diet. The Minnesota and Wisconsin wild rice regulations may be viewed as mainly protecting State industry economic concerns. However, the high price of wild rice makes the possibility of consumer fraud an issue.

Conclusions The high cost of wild rice makes this product prone to consumer deception through substitution and blending regardless of its relative market position compared with other rice products. **Therefore, the Committee suggests that FDA issue a formal advisory opinion or establish a common or usual name regulation defining wild rice in terms of its botanical name(s). Current State requirements should not be candidates for exemption from preemption until a formal FDA requirement is in place.**

LABELING OF ARTIFICIAL COLORINGS, FLAVORINGS, AND CHEMICAL PRESERVATIVES—SECTION 403(k)

FDCA Section 403(k) provides that a food is misbranded

if it bears or contains any artificial flavoring, artificial coloring, or chemical preservative, unless it bears labeling stating that fact: *Provided,* That to the extent that compliance with the requirements of this paragraph is impracticable, exemptions shall be established by regulation promulgated by the Secretary. The provisions of this paragraph and paragraphs (g) and (i) with respect to artificial coloring shall not apply in the case of butter, cheese, or ice cream. The provisions of this paragraph with respect to chemical preservatives shall not apply to a pesticide chemical when used in or on a raw agricultural commodity which is the produce of the soil.

Federal Requirements

The Pure Food and Drugs Act of 1906 first laid the statutory framework for regulation of artificial colorings, flavorings, and chemical preservatives. Section 7(4) of the 1906 Act declared that food was adulterated "if it be mixed, colored, powdered, coated, or stained in a manner whereby damage or inferiority is concealed." Section 7(5) deemed adulteration to include "any added poisonous or added deleterious ingredient which may render such article injurious to health." Preservatives were allowed as long as they could be removed prior to consumption. The 1906 Act did not require labeling of artificial coloring, flavorings, and chemical preservatives in foods.

FDCA, however, declared a food misbranded if its label did not declare the presence of artificial flavors, colors, and chemical preservatives. Congress acted further in this regard by twice amending the 1938 Act: in 1958, with the Food Additives Amendment (P.L. 85-929), and in 1960, with the Color Additive Amendments (P.L. 86-618). The former prohibited approval of any food additive if "the proposed use of the additive would promote deception of the consumer in violation of this chapter or would otherwise result in adulteration or in misbranding of food within the meaning of this chapter." Parallel language was contained in the Color Additive Amendments.

Current Requirements

FDA has established regulations that set out the rules on declaration of flavors, colorings, and preservatives (21 CFR §101.22). These regulations govern every aspect of the requirements established under FDCA Section 403(k), including applicable exemptions found at 21 CFR §101.100.

The definitions related to FDCA Section 403(k) are contained in 21 CFR §101.22(a)(1) and (2) through 21 CFR §101.22(a)(4). Artificial flavors include substances listed in 21 CFR §172.515(b) and §182.60, with spices listed in 21 CFR §182.10 and Part 184. Natural flavors include the natural essence or extractives obtained from plants listed in 21 CFR §172.510 and Part 184. The term "artificial color" means any color additive as defined in 21 CFR §70.3(f). A definition of chemical preservative is contained within 21 CFR §101.22(a)(5). A product's label must state that artificial colors, flavors, or chemical preservatives are present [21 CFR §101.22(a)(1)], and this message must be presented in a manner that can be understood by the consumer [21 CFR 101.22(a)(2)].

According to 21 CFR §101.22(b), foods subject to FDCA Section 403(k) require labeling "even though such food is not in package form." However, foods are exempt from compliance with Section 403(k) requirements when they are unpackaged and sold in small units [21 CFR §101.22(d)] whose labeling is not likely to be read "by the ordinary individual under customary conditions of purchase and use." Further, food sold in bulk is also exempt if the label for the bulk container is plainly in view or a counter sign is displayed that bears "prominently and conspicuously" the required information [21 CFR §101.22(e)]. Consistent with the language of Section 403(k), chemical preservatives applied to fruits and vegetables prior to harvest are also exempt from compliance [21 CFR §101.22(f)].

Foods that contain spices or natural and/or artificial flavors may declare those ingredients using generic terms rather than by their individual names. However, substances commonly understood to be foods (e.g., garlic powder, dehydrated onions, celery powder) must be declared by their common or usual name, as must salt (sodium chloride) and monosodium glutamate (MSG) [21 CFR §101.22(h)(3), (4)]. The use of words, pictures, or colors to indicate that a food contains a recognizable, characterizing flavor requires that the manufacturer declare such a flavor on the principal display panel in one of several means specified by the regulation [21 CFR §101.22(i)].

Chemical preservatives not exempted by 21 CFR §101.100 must be labeled with both the common or usual name of the ingredient and a separate identification of the function of the preservative [21 CFR §101.22(j)]. Certain color additives that are of health significance (e.g., that may cause allergic reactions) must be identified by their specific names [21 CFR Part 74 and 21 CFR §101.22(c)].

In 1986, FDA adopted a regulation limiting the use of sulfiting agents (21 CFR §182.3739 through §3862) but did not declare a preemptive policy. The agency stated that it would not preempt in the absence of a "genuine need to stop the proliferation of inconsistent requirements" (FDA, 1986). The existing FDA regulation states that sulfites must be declared on food labels if they are present above a given level. Below that level, they are considered an incidental additive and not required to be listed in the ingredient statement [21 CFR §101.100(a)(4)].

The Committee examined TC and administrative information letters regarding implementation, including specific interpretations of FDCA Section 403(k). There are several TC letters dating from 1940 that deal specifically with the determination that vanillin is an artificial flavoring and products (chocolate, in this case) containing it should be so labeled (TC-176, 1940). Likewise, caramel was determined to be an artificial color. Another TC letter details the methods of label declaration of its content (TC-203, 1940). During this period, nitrogen and carbon dioxide in canned foods were not considered chemical preservatives (TC-198, 1940).

In an information letter, the use of the words "color added" or "certified color added" was determined by FDA to be in compliance with FDCA Section 403(k) (Administrative Information Letter No. 87, 1949). With respect to label declarations of preservatives, the agency took the position in a 1963 Bureau of Enforcement Guideline that for finished foods in which flavorings such as spices have been treated with a chemical preservative, no label designating this practice is required if that chemical preservative was not intended to nor did it have any preservative effect on the finished food (BE-145, 1963). Active enforcement has occurred on labeling requirements for FD&C Yellow Dye No. 5 in foods has been active, due to the allergic reaction experienced by some consumers (21 CFR §74.705).

In a related section, FDCA Section 402(c) provides that a food is adulterated "if it is, or it bears or contains, a color additive which is unsafe" within the meaning of FDCA Section 706(a) dealing with certified or coal-tar colors.

Case Law

Two Federal court cases interpreting FDCA Section 403(k) in conjunction with other provisions of FDCA Section 403 were identified and reviewed. Neither provided extensive discussions of how the courts interpreted Section 403(k) and were valuable only as historical references. The Supreme Court concluded in *U.S. v. Sullivan*, 332 U.S. 689, 68 S.Ct. 331 (1948), that if a "violation . . . [is] a 'technical, innocent' one . . . for which the Administrator should have made an exemption," the criminal prosecution should be dropped. The United States District Court held that a taste test used to determine if squalene was added to a blend of olive and other vegetable oils was insufficient proof of misbranding under Section 403(k). The Second Circuit Court of Appeals reversed the decision on an adulteration charge but apparently supported the misbranding standard, *U.S. v. Antonio Corrao Corp.*, 185 F.2d 372, 375 (2d Cir.1950) (quoting district court opinion).

State Requirements

The statutes of 21 States are identical to Federal FDCA provisions but lack the exemption of butter, cheese, and ice cream from the required labeling of artificial coloring under FDCA Section 403(k). Other States differ from Federal law with respect to the labeling of flavorings, colorings, and preservatives in specific foods; they also differ in their labeling requirements for specific substances and the degree to which nonpackaged, bulk, and prepared foods should be labeled. These specific differences in State regulations, discovered in the materials made available to the Committee, are discussed below.

Label Requirements for Specific Colors, Flavors, or Preservatives

Connecticut requires that food to which a sulfiting agent has been added must be labeled with the name of the agent and its function [Conn. Stat. §21a-104(a)(2)]. Federal regulations implementing FDCA Section 403(k) require that sulfites be listed when present above the level of 10 parts per million [21 CFR §101.10(a)(4)].

Prohibitions on Colors, Flavors, and Chemical
Preservatives in Specific Foods

Minnesota regulations (Minn. Reg. §1550.0620) require that any "salad oil" be free of artificial coloration or added ingredients that cause it to appear "a shade of yellow"; the regulations also require that catsup and tomato sauces be free of added artificial color (Minn. Reg. §1550.0850). California prohibits the use of artificial colors or flavors in olive oil (Cal. Health & Safety Code §28481). A prohibition against artificial colors in vinegar exists in Rhode Island (R.I. Gen. Laws §21-22-1 and §21-22-3) and West Virginia (W.Va. Code §19-22-1, §19-22-5 and §19-22-6). Washington prohibits the use of yellow coloring in macaroni (Wash. Rev. Code §69.08.045).

The Pennsylvania State Code's Chapter 43, which governs food flavoring materials, states that it is unlawful to add color to vanilla or vanillin flavor and prohibits cider vinegar from containing artificial color (§9921-924).

Federal regulations require that artificial flavors, colors, or chemical preservatives be approved by FDA and declared on the label. FDCA Section 403(k) does not specifically prohibit the use of approved colors, flavors, or chemical preservatives in particular foods. It is not clear whether the State regulations noted above are "standards of identity" or States are attempting to prevent "economic adulteration." In any case, these statutes appear to require labeling "of the type" addressed by Section 403(k).

Label Requirements for Specific Foods Containing Artificial
Colorings, Flavorings, and Chemical Preservatives

Twenty-two States do not exempt butter and other dairy products from labeling requirements, in contrast to FDCA Section 403(k), which exempts butter, ice cream, and cheese from the required label declaration of colors, flavors, and chemical preservatives.[12]

---

[12] Alaska Stat. §17.20.040; Ariz. Rev. Stat. Ann. §36-906; Ark. Stat. Ann. §82-1111; Cal. Health & Safety Code §26559; Conn. Gen. Stat. §21a-102; Fla. Stat. §500.11; Ga. Code Ann. §26-2-28-11; Idaho Code §37-123; Kan. Stat. Ann. §28-21-11; Ky. Rev. Stat. Ann. §217.095; La. Rev. Stat. Ann. §608; Mass. 105 CMR §520.118; Mich. Comp. Laws §289.717; Minn. Stat. §33.03; N.H. Rev. Stat. Ann. §146.5; N.M. Stat. Ann. §25-2-11; N.D. Cent. Code §19-02.1-10; Ohio Rev. Code Ann. §3715.60; Okla. Stat. §63-1-1110; R.I. Gen. Laws §21-31-11; Vt. Stat. Ann. §4060; Wis. Stat §97.03.

Label Requirements Regarding Quantities of Artificial Colorings,
Flavorings, and Chemical Preservatives

Minnesota's regulations (Minn. Reg. §1550.0410) require that when two or more mixtures of preservatives are used, the names and percentages of each ingredient must be clearly printed in the order of predominance. They also require that the name and percentage of each ingredient used in oleomargarine be listed and its source revealed (Minn. Reg. §1550.0860). Ohio law requires that soft drink labels specify the name and amount of any preservative used (Ohio Rev. Code Ann. §913.24). Pennsylvania has a similar soft drink requirement (Pa. Stat. §790.7; §790.8). South Dakota requires that "[a]ll foods which contain any preservative, other than those substances specifically mentioned in §39-4-4, . . . shall be plainly and conspicuously labeled to show the presence and amount of such preservative" (S.D. Codified Laws Ann. §39-4-5). In contrast, Federal regulations currently do not require that the amount of the preservative used be specified on the label; however, they do require that the common name and function be listed.

Label Requirements for Colors, Flavors, or
Preservatives in Bulk Foods

Several States require that individual "bulk" foods be labeled regarding the use of a food coloring. Minnesota Regulation 1550.0870 requires that the color added to oranges not exceed the average representative natural color that the varietal oranges would have when naturally colored. Each orange and its container must be labeled "color added." California also requires that oranges sprayed with artificial coloring be labeled "color added" (Cal. Admin. Code Title 3, R. 365.3A). Texas requires all citrus fruits treated with "coloring matter" to be marked with the words "color added" (Tex. Agric. Code §95.011 and §95.012; §95.016 through §95.018). FDA only requires that a container or placard disclose the use of artificial coloring [21 CFR §101.22(e)].

Colorado requires the manufacturer of bulk foods sold at the retail level to label products as to the presence of any artificial color, flavor, or chemical preservative (Co. Stat. §25-4-1302). Likewise, Arizona statutes require that bulk foods offered self-service style to consumers include a declaration of artificial color or flavor and any chemical preservatives contained in the product (Ariz. Rev. Stat. Ann. §36-973).

Label Requirements for Foods Prepared and/or Served on Premises

Chapter 62, Section 23-62-1 of the Rhode Island Truth in Food Disclosure Law requires that a list of all preservatives and artificial ingredients added to food prepared on the premises of all retail preparers of food, including bakeries and restaurants, be available to consumers on request. Section 21a-104a of the Connecticut General Statutes applies to any bulk display of unpackaged foods, including those in a salad bar, offered for sale at any retail or wholesale establishment. The establishment is required to prominently display a sign warning that a particular product contains a sulfiting agent that may cause allergic reactions in some persons. Tennessee requires that food service establishments that treat produce with sulfiting agents post a sign stating that sulfites are used and list the items that are treated (Tenn. Code Ann. §53-8-116). West Virginia requires that hotels and restaurants that use sulfites on salad bars post a sign (W.Va. Code §16-6-22a.11).

Maine requires that food prepared at the retail level containing a crystalline form of MSG be labeled as such with the label either next to the nonpackaged food or the food as listed on the menu. Alternatively, the establishment can display a directory referring customers to information about the MSG content of unpackaged foods (Me. Rev. Stat. Ann. Title 22, §2157.13).

Other State Labeling Requirements

Two States require the labeling of chemicals used in seafood. For example, Maryland requires that each container of crabmeat contain information that a chemical is added (Md. Health-Gen. Code Ann. §21-339). Texas regulations on labeling crabmeat require a designation on the container if a chemical has been added (Texas Health & Safety Code §436.08).

Implementation

California claims that it has used its State labeling provisions with respect to artificial colors, flavors, and chemical preservatives in "repeated" and "successful" prosecution of violations to protect consumers from misbranded products (Sheneman, 1991). In general, however, States expressed concern with respect to their continuing ability to enforce existing

State regulations and uncertainty regarding their role in enforcement of Federal regulations.

Despite the differences between the Minnesota law cited above and Federal provisions, a letter to the Committee from that State expressed no concern about the loss of State laws to Federal preemption (Masso, 1991). Michigan expressed concern about a lack of clarity with respect to labeling of artificial colorings, flavorings, and chemical preservatives (Heffron, 1991). Generally, States with different or more stringent regulations for flavors, colors, and chemical preservatives believe that preemption under NLEA will reduce consumer protection in areas not now addressed by Federal statutes, regulations, or other implementing policies.

Industry Perspective

Industry comments indicate that most manufacturers consider FDA has adequately implemented the provisions of FDCA Section 403(k) for labeling artificial flavors, colors, and chemical preservatives (GMA, 1991). Given the complexity and detail of the implementing regulations that have evolved over 40 years, industry expressed the view that there is no reason for change.

Consumer Perspective

CSPI and other consumer groups represented at the Committee's public meeting stated that Federal regulation under FDCA Section 403(k) has been insufficient, citing Connecticut's sulfite labeling requirement as providing greater consumer and health protection than Federal requirements (CSPI/CNI/CFA/NCL, 1991). Connecticut requires that a sign be posted on bulk displays of unpackaged foods, such as salad bars, to indicate the presence of sulfites (Conn. Gen. Stat. §21a-1041). Such signs would inform consumers about foods that contain sulfiting agents, which can cause significant health effects in those sensitive to these chemicals. Some citizen petitions also indicated their belief that individual preservatives in foods should be declared on food labels (i.e., Clay, 1981).

The consumer representatives cited another example of State regulation related to FDCA Section 403(k) in which the Federal requirement is less stringent: the labeling of MSG when added to foods as an artificial flavor enhancer. While 21 CFR §101.22(h)(5) requires that MSG be identified by its common or usual name, other provisions of the Federal regulations create exceptions to this rule. Section §101.22(h)(1) permits the term "natural flavor" to be used for foods that contain up to 20 percent added

MSG. While such practices do not violate Federal regulations, consumers argue that those sensitive to MSG do not have the information they need to make informed purchasing decisions.

Conclusions

FDA regulations do not require that many added colors, flavors, and chemical preservatives be listed by their specific names on the ingredient listing but rather by generic names established for particular categories of ingredients. Thus, most flavors, colors, and spices need not necessarily be listed individually, which has been a long-standing source of debate between consumers and industry. Consumer groups argue that this type of generic labeling does not provide them with the information necessary to determine precisely the ingredients contained in a given product. On the other hand, more extensive labeling might crowd out other important information on the label. In addition, industry is reluctant to provide such information because it could reveal trade secrets. These arguments are now moot in regard to certified colors because NLEA requires that they be individually listed in the ingredient statement [NLEA Section 7(3)].

It appears that State requirements with respect to flavorings, colorings, and spices are frequently written in a way that combines the concepts of misbranding under FDCA Section 403(b) and economic adulteration under FDCA Section 402(b)(4). The latter section states that a food is adulterated if any substance has been added thereto or mixed or packed therewith so as to increase its bulk or weight, or reduce its quality or strength, or make it appear better or of greater value than it is. As a result, for many State labeling requirements for additives, colors, and chemical preservatives, there are not clear delineations among economic adulteration, health and safety issues, and misbranding requirements. It is clear, however, that State statutes and regulations that specifically address issues of adulteration, in contrast to misbranding, are not preempted under NLEA. This lack of preemption of adulteration provisions [NLEA Section 6(a)] would apply especially to any requirement respecting a warning statement in the labeling of food concerning the safety of the food or component of the food.

Before passage of NLEA, FDCA provided that colorings need not be declared by their common or usual name but could be designated by the collective term "colorings" [FDCA Sections 403(g) and (i)]. NLEA amended FDCA Section 403(g) with respect to colorings, so that after May 8, 1993, only colorings for which FDA does not require certification under FDCA Section 706(c) will be exempt from label declaration by their common or usual name. Although NLEA did not change the requirements for spices and flavoring or noncertified colors, FDA is encouraging firms to voluntarily declare spices by name when they are added to food. With respect to flavorings, the agency is continuing to support the exemption from required declaration, but voluntary declaration of noncertified coloring has been proposed (FDA, 1991a).

In the proposed 21 CFR §101.22(k) of June 21, 1991, the agency also recommended that manufacturers voluntarily declare all colorings in butter, cheese, and ice cream to provide consumers with more consistent information (FDA, 1991a). Further, the proposed regulations make clear that hypoallergenic foods and infant foods are subject to the labeling requirements of 21 CFR §105.62 and §105.65, which require the declaration by common or usual name of all ingredients including flavorings, colors, and spices.

The proposed 21 CFR §101.22(k) also deals with the labeling of protein hydrolysates used for flavor-related purposes. FDA's current regulations state that when the specified hydrolyzed vegetable proteins are used as ingredients in a fabricated food, they may be declared as "salt and hydrolyzed vegetable protein" (21 CFR §101.35). Moreover, the agency has stated that because protein hydrolysates are considered flavor enhancers and not flavorings, they must be declared by their common or usual name in the ingredient list when used in foods. Despite the existence of 21 CFR §101.35 and the agency's stated position, some manufacturers have taken the view that when protein hydrolysates are added to food as flavorings, they need not be declared by name in the ingredient list. Instead, these ingredients may be listed as flavor or natural flavor.

The agency has proposed to add a new Section (h)(7) to 21 CFR §101.22 to require that any protein hydrolysate used for flavor-related purposes in food be specifically declared in the ingredient list, because these ingredients function in foods both as flavors and flavor enhancers. In addition, because the source of a protein hydrolysate has a significant effect on its properties, inclusion of the source in the name is essential to meet the requirements of 21 CFR §102.5(a).

The agency also considered the potential for adverse reactions to glutamates and MSG, which are components of protein hydrolysates. Because MSG, as it occurs in protein hydrolysates, is a component of these ingredients and not itself an ingredient, it is not subject to the ingredient declaration requirement of FDCA. The agency does not believe that scientific evidence exists to establish that MSG causes particularly severe adverse reactions or support the claim that reactions that occur at low doses are life-threatening. Therefore, FDA has proposed—as a tentative decision—that it will not require the declaration of MSG in protein hydrolysates

(FDA, 1991). The Committee is aware that the labeling of glutamate is a safety issue and not preempted under NLEA.

The requirements of Section 6(a)(2) and Section 7 of NLEA will have a direct impact on the requirements of FDCA Section 403(k) and parallel State requirements. However, in light of the proposed regulatory changes to 21 CFR §101.22, and FDCA Section 402(c) on adulteration is not preempted by NLEA (health-related warnings are exempt from preemption), many issues addressed by specific State regulations will either be covered by the proposed implementing rules or not be subject to preemption under NLEA.

The concerns of the consumer representatives reflect a mixture of safety and misbranding issues and may represent a need for additional statutory authority and enforcement (Chapter 6). To the extent possible, FDA should provide guidance to States and industry in determining whether a State requirement is related to FDCA Section 403(k) or a requirement under the State adulteration provisions, with respect to "health-related" warnings.

Based on its analysis, criteria, and current FDA regulatory activity, the Committee concludes that FDCA Section 403(k) is adequately implemented. The Committee further concludes that State labeling requirements related to FDCA Section 403(k) are candidates for preemption.

REFERENCES

AARP (American Association of Retired Persons). 1986. Truth About Aging: Guidelines for Accurate Communications. Washington, D.C.: AARP.

AFDO (Association of Food and Drug Officials). 1984. Uniform State Bottled Water Code. York, Pa.: AFDO.

AFDO (Association of Food and Drug Officials). 1991. Statement of R.D. Sowards, Jr., AFDO, at the Public Meeting of the Committee on State Food Labeling, Food and Nutrition Board, Institute of Medicine, Washington, D.C. May 30.

Clay, N. 1981. Citizen petition to the Food and Drug Administration, no. 81P-0330. October 12, 1981. Rockville, Md.:Dockets Management Branch, FDA.

Crawford, B., Florida Department of Agriculture and Consumer Services. 1991. Letter to the Committee on State Food Labeling, Food and Nutrition Board, Institute of Medicine, Washington, D.C. July 5.

CSPI/CNI/CFA/NCL (Center for Science in the Public Interest, Community Nutrition Institute, Consumer Federation of America, and the National Consumers League). 1991. Statement of Sharon Lindan, Assistant Director for Legal Affairs, CSPI, on behalf of CSPI/CNI/CFA/NCL at the Public Meeting of the Committee on State Food Labeling, Food and Nutrition Board, Institute of Medicine, Washington, D.C. May 30.

Davis, C.F., Maine Department of Agriculture. 1991. Letter to the Committee on State Food Labeling, Food and Nutrition Board, Institute of Medicine, Washington, D.C. Sept. 3.

Dunsmore, G.M., Vermont Department of Agriculture. 1991. Letter to the Committee on State Food Labeling, Food and Nutrition Board, Institute of Medicine, Washington, D.C. July 15.

Englender, S.J., Arizona Department of Health Services. 1991. Letter to the Committee on State Food Labeling, Food and Nutrition Board, Institute of Medicine, Washington, D.C. July 9.

Eskin, S.B., Public Policy Consultant. 1991. Letter to the Committee on State Food Labeling, Food and Nutrition Board, Institute of Medicine, Washington, D.C. Dec. 5.

FDACS (Florida Department of Agriculture and Consumer Services). 1991. Statement of Bob Crawford, Commissioner, FDACS, at the Public Meeting of the Committee on State Food Labeling, Food and Nutrition Board, Institute of Medicine, Washington, D.C. May 30.

FDACS/FDC (Florida Department of Agriculture and Consumer Services and Florida Department of Citrus). 1991. Memoranda outlining the impact of national uniform food labeling on the Florida Citrus Code. March 25 and Oct. 15.

FDA (Food and Drug Administration). 1973a. Bottled Water; Proposed Quality Standards. Fed. Reg 38:1019–1020; Jan. 8.

FDA (Food and Drug Administration). 1973b. Food Labeling; Imitation; Proposed Rule. Fed. Reg. 38:2138–2139; Jan. 19.

FDA (Food and Drug Administration). 1975. Quality Standards for Bottled Water; Final Rule. Fed. Reg. 40:21932–21934, May 20.

FDA (Food and Drug Administration). 1983. Food Labeling; Use of the Term Imitation; Proposed Rule Related. Fed. Reg. 48:37665–37666; Aug. 19.

FDA (Food and Drug Administration). 1988. The Fish List—FDA Guide to Acceptable Market Names for Food Fish Sold in Interstate Commerce. Washington, D.C.: Government Printing Office.

FDA (Food and Drug Administration). 1991a. Food Labeling; Declaration of Ingredients; Proposed Rule. Fed. Reg. 56:28591–28636; June 21.

FDA (Food and Drug Administration). 1991b. Food Labelin; Declaration of Ingredients; Common or Usual Name for Nonstandardized Foods; Diluted Juice Beverages; Proposed Rule. Fed. Reg. 56:30452–30466; July 2.

Frank, R.L., Olsson, Frank and Weeda, P.C. 1991. Letter to the Committee on State Food Labeling, Food and Nutrition Board, Institute of Medicine, Washington, D.C. Oct. 16.

GMA (Grocery Manufacturers of America). 1991. Statement of Sherwin Gardner, Vice President, Science and Technology, GMA, at the Public Meeting of the Committee on State Food Labeling, Food and Nutrition Board, Institute of Medicine, Washington, D.C. May 30.

Harris, A. 1983. Growers in Valdalia savor the sweet success of their onions. Washington Post p. a16. July 3.

Heffron, E.C., Michigan State Department of Agriculture. 1991. Letter to the Committee on State Food Labeling, Food and Nutrition Board, Institute of Medicine, Washington, D.C. July 11.

Hutt, P.B. 1987. Development of Federal law regulating slack fill and deceptive packaging of food, drugs, and cosmetics. Food Drug Cosmetic Law J. 42:1–37.

Hutt, P.B. 1989. Regulating the misbranding of food. Food Technol. 43(9):288–295.

Hutt, P.B., and Merrill, R.A. 1991. Food and Drug Law: Cases and Materials. 2nd ed. Westbury, N.Y.: Foundation Press.

KGF (Kraft General Foods). 1991. Statement of Merrill S. Thompson, Special Counsel, Arnold & Porter, at the Public Meeting of the Committee on State Food Labeling, Food and Nutrition Board, Institute of Medicine, Washington, D.C. May 30.

Lindan, S., Assistant Director for Legal Affairs, Center for Science in the Public Interest. 1991. Letter to the Committee on State Food Labeling, Food and Nutrition Board, Institute of Medicine, Washington, D.C. July 5.

Lorman, A.J. 1990. Food standards and the quest for healthier foods. Pp. 320-342 in Nutrition Labeling: Issues and Directions for the 1990s. Report of the Committee on the Nutrition

Components of Food Labeling, Food and Nutrition Board, Institute of Medicine. Washington, D.C.: National Academy Press.

Masso, T.W., Minnesota Department of Agriculture. 1991. Letter to the Committee on State Food Labeling, Food and Nutrition Board, Institute of Medicine, Washington, D.C. Sept. 10.

McClellan, D., Utah State Department of Agriculture. 1991. Letter to the Committee on State Food Labeling, Food and Nutrition Board, Institute of Medicine, Washington, D.C. July 8.

Nebe, J.L., Nevada State Department of Human Resources. 1991. Letter to the Committee on State Food Labeling, Food and Nutrition Board, Institute of Medicine, Washington, D.C. July 3.

NFERF (National Fisheries Education and Research Foundation). 1991a. Position on Use of FDA Compliance Policy for Naming Seafood Products. Washington, D.C.: NFERF.

NFERF (National Fisheries Education and Research Foundation). 1991b. The Retail Seafood Identity System. Washington, D.C.: Government Printing Office.

NFPI (National Frozen Pizza Institute). 1991. Statement of Eugene Welka, President, NFPI, at the Public Meeting of the Committee on State Food Labeling, Food and Nutrition Board, Institute of Medicine, Washington, D.C. May 30.

Niles, R., Georgia Department of Agriculture. 1991a. Letter to the Committee on State Food Labeling, Food and Nutrition Board, Institute of Medicine, Washington, D.C. June 17.

Niles, R., Georgia Department of Agriculture. 1991b. Letter to the Committee on State Food Labeling, Food and Nutrition Board, Institute of Medicine, Washington, D.C. Sept. 24.

NDMA (Nonprescription Drug Manufacturers Association). 1990. Voluntary Codes and Guidelines of the OTC [Over the Counter] Medicines Industry. Washington, D.C.: NDMA.

NDMA (Nonprescription Drug Manufacturers Association). 1991. Label Readability Guidelines. Washington, D.C.: NDMA.

Otwell, W.S. 1985. Florida Seafood Regulations and Regulators. Florida Seagrant College Program, Report No. 72. Gainesville, Fla. University of Florida.

Prakash, S. 1991. Looking to ride a bottled water wave. Washington Post Business, March 16. p. 3.

Quaker Oats and Schreiber Foods. 1991. Statement of Richard L. Frank, Partner, Olsson, Frank and Weeda, P.C., on behalf of the Quaker Oats Company and Schreiber Foods, Inc., at the Public Meeting of the Committee on State Food Labeling, Food and Nutrition Board, Institute of Medicine, Washington, D.C. May 30.

Rudd, J., Arizona Consumers Council. 1991. Letter to the Committee on State Food Labeling, Food and Nutrition Board, Institute of Medicine, Washington, D.C. July 15.

Schaffer, G., Connecticut State Department of Consumer Protection. 1991. Letter to the Committee on State Food Labeling, Food and Nutrition Board, Institute of Medicine, Washington, D.C. May 28.

Senger, K., South Dakota Department of Health. 1991. Letter to the Committee on State Food Labeling, Food and Nutrition Board, Institute of Medicine, Washington, D.C. July 8.

Shank, F.R. Director, Center for Food Safety and Applied Nutrition, Food and Drug Administration. 1991. Testimony of Fred R. Shank before the Subcommittee on Oversight and Investigations, House Committee on Energy and Commerce, U.S. Congress. April 10.

Sheneman, J.M., California Department of Health Services. 1991. Letter to the Committee on State Food Labeling, Food and Nutrition Board, Institute of Medicine, Washington, D.C. July 12.

State Attorneys General. 1991. Statement of Attorneys General of the States of California, Iowa, Minnesota, Missouri, New York, Texas, and Wisconsin to the Committee on State Food Labeling, Food and Nutrition Board, Institute of Medicine, Washington, D.C. May 30.

Tamura, M., Hawaii State Department of Health. 1991. Letter to the Committee on State Food Labeling, Food and Nutrition Board, Institute of Medicine, Washington, D.C. June 27.

Van Wagner, L.R. 1991. Crackdown on misleading labels. Food Processing 52(3):8-12.

Wiesenberger, A. 1991. The pocket guide to bottled water. Contemporary Books, Chicago, Ill.

Woodward, B. 1991. Presentation by Betsy Woodward, Chief, Food Laboratory, Division of Chemistry, Florida Department of Agriculture and Consumer Services, before the Committee on State Food Labeling, Food and Nutrition Board, Institute of Medicine, Washington, D.C. July 30.

6

Issues Raised by States, Consumers, and Industry

The charge to the Committee was to consider the adequacy of the Food and Drug Administration's (FDA) implementation of six provisions of Section 403 of the Food, Drug, and Cosmetic Act of 1938, as amended (FDCA), to determine whether State requirements of similar character should be preempted. There are two important changes in the legal environment that forms the context of this inquiry. The first change is that Congress has mandated a comprehensive and undoubtedly costly revamping of food labels to provide improved nutrition and other information on food products for consumers. The second change, as part of this requirement for new information, is that Congress has decided that States should no longer continue to enforce certain local food labeling requirements that are different from those of other States and/or the Federal government. The Nutrition Labeling and Education Act (NLEA) spoke clearly on uniformity (i.e., only one set of rules) and preemption (i.e., that those rules should be Federal). However, the Act also allowed States a role in both shaping (i.e., through the petition process) and enforcing those rules.

In the information obtained from States, localities, food and drug officials, and industry and consumer groups, the Committee received many comments on issues that were not directly related to its specific charge under NLEA. The Committee felt, however, that these issues were germane to the issue of uniform food labeling regulation and devoted considerable discussion to their significance in relation to the central topics of the study. As appropriate, these issues were taken into consideration in the discussion of the specific sections under study (Chapter 5). The Committee agreed that these issues should be of concern to FDA and has therefore included this discussion as part of its report. The various conflicting views are presented without evidence or examples because, in general, none were provided to the Committee.

As part of its information-gathering activities, the Committee asked State and local officials and consumer groups to comment on the six questions that appear in Appendix C. One of those questions concerned whether there were any other issues that respondents believed should be brought to the Committee's attention as it deliberated on the adequacy of implementation of FDCA and preemption of State requirements. In response to this question, the following points were raised as being of major concern to respondents, although they recognized that these issues were beyond the specific charge of the Committee:

- The adequacy of the fiscal and personnel resources applied by FDA in enforcing its food labeling requirements as a dimension of implementation.
- The importance of the enforcement activities of the States to ensure consumer protection in the area of food labeling.
- The value of existing cooperative relationships between FDA and the States, which have been developed and strengthened over many years.
- The concerns of States about FDA's implementation of the petition process of NLEA for exemption of a State requirement from preemption and State enforcement of Federal requirements, so that these processes will be uncomplicated and well managed.

The importance of these issues was reiterated through a variety of communications from professional food and drug regulatory groups, food companies, trade associations, and national consumer organizations. An additional issue of particular concern to the food industry was the economic cost of nonuniformity and the potential savings to be realized through increased national uniform food labeling.

ENFORCEMENT AS A DIMENSION OF IMPLEMENTATION

Many State officials and a number of consumer groups commented on the importance of enforcement and the future role of the States under NLEA. Commissioner Bob Crawford of the Florida Department of Agriculture and Consumer Services identified a number of problems in his letter to the Committee:

> The states are the foot soldiers in the area of food labeling review and enforcement and must be included as equal partners in implementation and enforcement. The states are the crucibles from which good national legislation in consumer issues

evolves. To provide total preemption that negates this extremely valuable function will be a disservice to the consumers of this nation. State legislators are not likely to fund state food programs in labeling unless they feel that the state has a voice and that the constituency's best interest will be served. It is critical that preemption not go beyond setting national standards and it is essential that there be a mechanism for states, with justifiable reason, to have a different standard. It is also crucial that the states be involved as full partners in developing any new standards (Crawford, 1991, p. 5).

Betty Harden of the Maryland Division of Food Control also identified enforcement as critical to any successful implementation of NLEA.

There were several differing opinions offered by the speakers and what seemed to me to be some worthwhile suggestions. However, the most important element in the implementation formula which I did not hear mentioned, is enforcement. If the Congressional intent of its charge to the Committee was to confine the determination of adequacy to assessing whether the Food and Drug Administration had promulgated the necessary regulations, then the real measure of adequate implementation will be overlooked and the determination will be superficial and based solely on a paper exercise. I would submit that fulfillment of the common goal of ensuring a safe and wholesome food supply demands enforcement and the degree of enforcement hinges on the availability of resources (Harden, 1991, p. 2).

The Association of Food and Drug Officials' (AFDO) statement to the Committee commented favorably on the recent enforcement actions taken by FDA but expressed concern about what it perceived as FDA's recent history of inaction. AFDO reflected the view held by the State and local regulatory officials who are its members:

The recent actions taken by the new FDA Commissioner David Kessler to crack down on deceptive food labeling have not gone unnoticed by AFDO. We commend the actions as both necessary and correct. However, as state officials we are also very much aware of the lack of enforcement *and* lack of "adequacy" of federal regulations which have resulted in the current state of affairs with respect to food labeling. It would be correct to assume that neither the states nor the state attorneys general would have become so involved in food labeling on a national level had it not been for the lack of federal enforcement. It would also be accurate to say that Congress would not have enacted the NLEA if the FDA had adequately enforced its regulations and had adopted new regulations as needed. The Office of Management and Budget further impeded the process by its inactivity with regard to newly proposed regulations (Sowards, 1991a, p. 4).

In the May 1991 *Final Report of the Advisory Committee on the Food and Drug Administration*, that Committee's Food Subcommittee recognized the key role enforcement plays in the implementation of the law and a vigorous FDA is the most effective deterrent to the adoption of diverse and inconsistent State requirements. The Subcommittee also indicated that FDA has not been a vigorous enforcer over the past decade (DHHS, 1991). The Advisory Committee further stated that:

> . . . from its inception FDA has focused heavily on law enforcement. . . . The ability to detect violations of the law and deal with them vigorously and swiftly is central to the Agency's credibility. . . . Recent events have raised doubts about the FDA's current capacity to conduct effective law enforcement. . . . Another feature of the enforcement landscape that deserves notice is the need for priority setting in light of resource shortfalls. It is well known, for example, that the Agency has for several years largely abandoned efforts to combat economic deception in the sale of food and cosmetics choosing appropriately to allocate depleted resources to safety related violations (DHHS, 1991, p. 25–27).

The comments made to this Committee reflect the fact that FDA's choice to direct priorities and enforcement actions toward health and safety violations first is not unfamiliar to State officials. States generally have understood the problems that FDA has faced in terms of continually reduced resources. Fortunately, and frequently, the combined resources of both Federal and State offices have been utilized to correct economic, as well as health and safety, violations. The Advisory Committee recognized the value of such cooperation and recommended that FDA develop programs to restore confidence, enlisting the continued cooperation of the States. The report further recommended new actions to be taken if FDA is to succeed in accomplishing the heavy responsibility NLEA has placed on an already beleaguered, understaffed agency (DHHS, 1991).

STATE ACTION UNDER NLEA

In the administrative process established by NLEA, Federal preemption is not intended to leave the States powerless, because they are provided with the opportunity to petition for exemption from preemption and enforce Federal requirements. State officials have raised some serious concerns, however, about how the procedure will work. NLEA Section 4, entitled "State Enforcement," outlined the process the States and FDA must follow if a State action is to be undertaken. NLEA allows a State to bring civil enforcement proceedings within its own jurisdiction or restrain violations of any labeling provisions if the food is subject to the proceedings of that State. Such proceedings, however, are not to be commenced (1) until 30 days after the State has notified FDA of its intention to begin such a proceeding, (2) before 90 days if the Secretary has commenced an informal or formal enforcement action pertaining to the food, or (3) if the Secretary is diligently prosecuting a case in court pertaining to such food or has settled such a case or enforcement action.

Comments made during Senate debate on the bill supported the need of a State to be able to act on behalf of its constituents. In his statement, Senator Metzenbaum emphasized that:

The first matter involves the subject of preemption. We want to clarify that nothing in Section 4 of the bill, as amended, prevents a State from acting under law to address an emergency.

It is also important that this program, which requires nationally uniform nutritional labeling, is sensitive to the regulatory roles played by the States. This bill has been refined to provide national uniformity where it is most necessary, while otherwise preserving State regulatory authority where it is appropriate (U.S. Congress, 1990, p. 16609).

A review of the comments submitted to the Committee revealed that there are differing opinions on the exact intent of the language of NLEA Section 4. Correspondence from AFDO's Food Labeling Committee raised a question concerning whether NLEA requires a State to give FDA 30 days' notice before the State undertakes an enforcement action under FDCA (AFDO, 1991). This question suggests confusion on the part of some State officials. NLEA clearly requires States to give FDA 30 days' notice before taking action under an FDCA provision.

In their response to the Committee, some consumer groups predicted problems for those States without laws identical to the Federal provisions. The groups noted that even though States have the authority to enforce the Federal statute, the procedural process, involving FDA notification and the required delay of State agencies (in deference to Federal enforcement) until FDA replies, will place a strain on the financial and investigative resources of the States. Concern was expressed that there would be less State initiative in this area because of the required notification and the 30-day response period (Lindan, 1991).

In a letter to the Committee, the Grocery Manufacturers of America (GMA) maintained that, by following correct procedures, States retain power to enforce a food labeling matter in a State court as long as the States are enforcing State provisions that are identical to the six designated Sections (Gardner and Guarino, 1991). Furthermore, in situations in which only intrastate commerce is involved, FDA has no jurisdiction, and State laws and regulations are not preempted.

The importance of this section being clarified by FDA is reflected in the opinions expressed by two attorneys experienced in food law. When asked whether NLEA required a State to give FDA 30 days' notice before undertaking an enforcement action under its own statute or regulations, George Burditt (Partner, Burditt, Bowles & Radzius, Chartered) responded to the question with an unequivocal no. He stated that NLEA Section 4 authorizes States to enforce the Federal act if the food is located in that

State and requires States to notify the Federal government only if they intend to enforce the Federal law; it makes no comment about the State law. Burditt pointed out that States have the right to enforce their own laws on labeling and denial of that right would be a "perfectly clear violation of the federalism system of our government if a State couldn't act to enforce its own laws without giving the Federal government 30 days notice" (Burditt, 1991).

In response to Burditt's position, Merrill Thompson (Partner, Arnold & Porter) agreed that a State may be unrestrained in its application of the law to intrastate commerce but that it is still just on the team in relation to interstate commerce. Thompson maintains that since NLEA gives the States total access to the Federal law and regulations, it is only logical "that the Congressional insistence on identical State requirements be understood to require the States to tie their implementation processes to the Federal processes including enforcement" (Thompson, 1991).

Because of the apparent confusion over how NLEA Section 4 is to be implemented, the Committee welcomed the proposed regulations on State enforcement under NLEA, which were published by FDA on November 27, 1991 (FDA, 1991b). The proposed regulations outlined the procedures that States should follow in taking enforcement action. Beginning on November 8, 1992, States are authorized under NLEA to bring action on certain misbranding violations of FDCA in Federal court to supplement FDA's enforcement activities. A State's ability to exercise this new authority to enforce Federal law is predicated on certain conditions:

1. A proceeding may not be commenced unless that State has given notice to FDA that it intends to bring such proceeding and waits 30 days after giving notice to institute action.
2. After receiving notice, FDA has 30 days to commence an informal or formal enforcement action pertaining to the food in question, and if it does so, the State may not bring its proceeding until an additional 60 days have passed.
3. Where FDA is actively prosecuting the case in court, has settled it, or settled the informal or formal enforcement action pertaining to the food, the State may not institute a proceeding.

In the proposed regulation, FDA has interpreted informal enforcement actions to include Warning Letters, recalls, and detentions, which can all be taken administratively; formal action has been interpreted to involve seizures, injunctions, and prosecutions, which require initiation of judicial proceedings. The proposed regulation also delineates the procedures that a State must follow in notifying the agency of its intention to institute an enforcement action, including a standard format and information for the letter of notification, signed by a State official authorized to institute the proposed action. In addition, the agency has proposed the procedures it will follow in responding to a State's notification to ensure that the State knows the status of the agency's intent concerning the State's proposed action. FDA has stated its belief that an FDA action anywhere in the country against the food in question would bar a State action against the food in Federal court. The agency notes, however, that provisions of NLEA do not preclude State enforcement under its own identical statute or regulations in State court (FDA, 1991b).

All concerned parties should have commented on the proposed regulations on State enforcement procedures (by the February 25, 1992 deadline). FDA will need to follow implementation of these requirements closely to allow the States to play an effective role in enforcement. Concomitantly, although NLEA and the proposed regulations do not require FDA notification for a State to take action under its own statutes and regulations in a State court, it seems reasonable, in the interest of the goals of national uniformity and cooperation, that some mechanism should be established for States to apprise FDA and other States of actions taken in State courts.

COOPERATIVE RELATIONSHIPS BETWEEN FDA AND THE STATES

It is also important that FDA and the States enhance the mechanisms available for cooperative working relationships. Open communication channels are needed to address emerging issues on a regular basis. Active dialogue to handle issues before they are either addressed by one jurisdiction or the petition process will allow for early input from State regulators in the development of Federal responses to these emerging issues.

In recent years, the States and FDA have jointly planned their programs to "effectively utilize their combined minimal resources to obtain maximum results" (Wilms, 1991a). State programs have augmented those of FDA and extended consumer protection beyond what the Federal government alone could provide. In a speech to the American Legislative Exchange Council in April 1989, then FDA Commissioner Frank E. Young stressed the importance of cooperative efforts among FDA and State and local officials to ensure consumer protection, given the great challenges to be faced with limited resources. In underlining the importance of these relationships, he recalled the words of President Theodore Roosevelt: "How much good for the whole people results from the hearty cooperation of the federal and state officials in securing a given reform . . . there must be the closest cooperation between the national and state governments in administering these laws" (Young, 1989).

In his comments to the Committee, Heinz Wilms, FDA's Director of Federal-State Relations, noted that Federal and State officials, along with support from the regulated industry, have worked for many years "to establish uniform legal codes on which to base enforcement procedures." He highlighted a number of initiatives and programs that are funded or supported by FDA and aimed at promoting uniform procedures:

- Joint FDA/State inspections
- Regional and district conferences
- FDA formal training courses
- Communication systems such as NRSTEN (National, Regional, and State Telecommunications Network)
- Coordinated Operations Plan for Emergencies (COPE)
- State contract program

Wilms concluded that "the continuation of these State and Federal cooperative efforts is important to the enforcement of the statute. The passage of NLEA hopefully will not weaken the States' resolve to be a strong participant and partner in the process of implementing that law" (Wilms, 1991b).

In comments received by the Committee, State officials and consumer groups generally agreed that Federal preemption under NLEA is unlikely to be accompanied or followed by major new FDA funding to allow the agency to increase its regulatory efforts to make up for a perceived decrease in State regulatory efforts because of preempted requirements. They express concern that State legislatures that are anxious to find cost-saving measures may redirect the appropriations for food labeling regulation to other State programs, resulting in a decrease in consumer protection. Many State officials fear this elimination of State-funded programs and are skeptical about the future of enforcement, the subsequent implementation of the statute, and, ultimately, consumer protection (i.e., Corbin, 1991; Crawford, 1991; Harden, 1991; Lindan, 1991; Masso, 1991, McClellan, 1991; Niles, 1991; Rudd, 1991; Sevchik, 1991; Sowards, 1991b).

It is not yet possible to predict the possible loss of State resources, participation, and involvement in the food regulation scheme set into motion by NLEA. State food regulation programs address both misbranding and adulteration activities without delineating the amount of funds spent in each area. The importance of States' efforts in food safety regulation, which was not changed by NLEA, suggests that there could be relatively little decrease in total State funding of food regulation activities. Only future events will provide the answer to those who have expressed concerns. Meanwhile, both Federal and State officials have emphasized that cooperation, and sharing of responsibilities and programs, should be both continued and enhanced (Crawford, 1991; Heffron 1991; Sevchik, 1991; Wilms, 1991a).

PREEMPTION AND THE PETITION PROCESS

In general, consumer groups who provided comments to the Committee are opposed to the preemption of State and local laws by the Federal government. In their responses, these groups argued that State and local governmental bodies can react more quickly and effectively than Federal agencies to protect consumers. In addition, they can encourage the Federal government to improve national standards and address newly emerging issues. Consumer groups have thus called for an expeditious petitioning process that would allow States wide latitude in exemptions from preemption under NLEA to protect consumers (CSPI/CNI/CFA/NCL, 1991).

One principle of particular importance expressed by the consumer groups is the right of citizens to have State and local governments that are responsive to their needs. In support of this view, they cited a recent article in which Bruce Silverglade of the Center for Science in the Public Interest argued that "[s]tates should be free to address local concerns in a manner they believe is appropriate. The ability to address local needs is especially appropriate because state officials are often closer to the people they are trying to serve than the officials in Washington, D.C." (Silverglade, 1990, p. 145).

Another group, Public Voice for Food and Health Policy, took the position that preemption has the potential to drain innovation and vigor from the consumer protection system. One result of such a drain would be that future marketing schemes that hurt consumers would be left largely unchallenged (Haas, 1991). Using examples from different areas of regulation in support of their positions, especially food safety, the consumer groups emphasized the importance of vigorous State and local action in the national consumer protection regime.

Although few consumer groups cited specific protection that would be jeopardized under the NLEA food labeling preemption provisions, all pointed out that the role of the State agencies in responding to emerging issues in food labeling could be curtailed by preemption. In their view, limits on the States' role might hasten the obsolescence of Federal policies by preventing regulatory innovation; they might also hamper the ability of States to enforce current Federal law and directly undermine the policy objectives set forth in NLEA (Haas, 1991; Lindan, 1991; Mitchell, 1990).

The Committee believes that FDA's rules must take into account genuine local needs that are based on evidence to justify preemption or exemption of State requirements.

A background paper prepared for the Committee reviewed the recommendations of a report on the petition process prepared by the National Food Processors Association (NFPA, 1991) and commented on the State petition process in general (Bryson, 1991). The paper concluded that the petition process could be a workable procedure but predicted that it would neither be expedient nor easy to implement.

One NFPA recommendation suggested that the procedural provisions in 16 CFR Part 1061 [Consumer Product Safety Commission (CPSC)] could provide the basis for similar provisions that FDA could adopt to implement NLEA Section 403A(b). The Bryson paper concluded that this suggestion had merit despite the difficulties experienced by States in providing "adequate" information to enable CPSC to act on their requests. Bryson urged FDA to require only necessary and reasonable information and specify the criteria that will be used to grant or deny an exemption request. The paper suggests that it is incumbent on FDA not to arbitrarily require further information if it is clear that the State submission has met the stated requirements; in addition, the agency should work diligently to finalize its decision on a State exemption request within 180 days after receipt of the request. The paper concluded that, ideally, FDA, industry, consumers, and the State should work together to develop the regulation that specifies the information to be provided in a State preemption exemption request.

The NFPA study also recommended that the CPSC regulation (16 CFR §1061.9) pertaining to the burden on interstate commerce be incorporated into FDA regulations. The Bryson paper emphasized, however, that the decision to exempt a State from preemption must be based primarily on issues of consumer protection and concerns about overburdening interstate commerce should be of secondary importance.

With respect to NLEA Section 403A(b)(3), which states that the State requirement must be designed to address a particular need for information that is not met by the FDCA requirement, NFPA suggested that if a State does, in fact, demonstrate that a particular need is not met by Federal law, FDA must propose an amendment of its regulation to meet that need, rather than authorize a State exemption from preemption. The Bryson paper concluded that the position taken by NFPA is particularly meritorious. The paper specifically noted that FDA must be alert to recognize instances in which States have identified a regulatory need that has nationwide implications and it should move promptly to propose Federal adoption. Bryson also provided the following suggestions and conclusions:

- Requests for exemption should be reviewed by an advisory panel that includes at least one State agency representative.
- States must actively participate in the new Federal process. States may decline to participate, but if they do, they run the chance of losing even more than the preemption established by NLEA. FDA is urged to work with the States, solicit their input, utilize the committee process, develop models, and establish an office in the Center for Food Safety and Applied Nutrition to receive and assist in finalizing State submissions.
- Organizations of food and drug officials will need to take an active role in representing the States on NLEA matters. The paper supported an AFDO request that FDA designate a specific staff person in the Division of Federal-State Relations as a single point source of information on NLEA for State regulatory agencies (Bryson, 1991, pp. 12-13).

On November 27, 1991, FDA published a proposed regulation for the petition process concerned with preemption of State requirements. For any State statute or regulation that will be preempted under the provisions of NLEA, the petition process serves as a mechanism by which States can request FDA to exempt them from the effective dates for preemption of a specific State provision. Under this proposal, if a State submits a petition for exemption from Federal preemption under NLEA Section 403A(b) by May 8, 1992, the State requirement will not be preempted until after November 8, 1992, or FDA acts on the petition—whichever is later. (FDA, 1991b) The State requirement must meet three criteria to be granted an exemption: it must (1) not cause any food to be in violation of any applicable requirement under Federal law; (2) not unduly burden interstate commerce; and (3) address a particular need for information that has not been met by the existing requirements of Federal law. The petition must also

- identify and document the State requirement for which exemption is sought;
- identify the Federal requirement that is believed to preempt the State requirement;
- describe the rationale of the State requirement and compare it with the Federal requirement;
- address with specificity the grounds for exemption from preemption stated in NLEA; and
- discuss the particular information need that the State requirement is designed to meet that is not met by the Federal law.

Also required is a claim for categorical exclusion of an environmental assessment, identification of the person and address to be notified, and a certification by the petitioner that the petition includes all information and views relied on in its development.

Under the proposed regulations, FDA would provide one of three responses to the petitioner within 90 days:

1. the agency tentatively determines that the petition merits the granting of an exemption and intends to publish a proposed regulation to grant exemption in the *Federal Register*;
2. the agency denies the petition and states the reasons for such denial; or
3. the agency provides a tentative response stating why it has been unable to reach a decision on the petition.

Exemptions would be granted only to the petitioner State. If the issue is national in scope, FDA would consider amending the Federal requirement. In proposing its regulations on exemption from preemption, FDA relied in part on the policy in Executive Order 12612 on federalism, "that preemption of State law shall be restricted to the minimum level necessary to achieve the objectives of the statute." As a corollary to this proposition, FDA stated that exemption from preemption should be liberally granted in line with statutory objectives (FDA, 1991b).

As proposed, the petition process provides a mechanism by which States can address their particular needs both before preemption takes effect and afterward, should the need arise. Hawaii's labeling requirement for poi is a case in point. The Committee understands the need of consumers in Hawaii to have such protection when purchasing a product of historical importance to local cultural and ethnic needs. This type of importance and history of use could most certainly be supported by the State through citations to its published literature, annual sales figures, demographic data, and other similar sources. The Committee believes it is important for States to use this mechanism to deal with their particular local needs and unanticipated future issues that may be national in scope but yet have not been addressed by FDA. The petition process or other mechanisms should also allow States to suggest those instances in which they believe some informational requirements may be considered candidates for Federal adoption. In this way, the States may still serve as the front line of consumer protection that they have been in the past. For its part, FDA must ensure that the process' requirements for information are clear to the States and follow its own time schedule for action on petitions. The agency needs to make decisions as rapidly as possible and not use a tentative response of "unable to make a decision" (item no. 3 above) to place a State on hold for months. FDA also should use petitions as a way to evaluate its own activities in regard to adequate implementation of the various misbranding provisions of FDCA.

ECONOMIC IMPACT OF NONUNIFORMITY

One of the issues that industry representatives continued to raise was the substantial costs entailed in nonuniform State food labeling requirements. Although most costs could be expressed as dollar amounts, the managerial frustrations associated with nonuniformity cannot and should not be discounted. In pursuing this issue, the Committee was advised by industry that the economic impact of nonuniformity of Federal and State requirements for food labeling is very significant and under extreme conditions can be tremendous.

The Committee questioned nine food companies and two trade associations on the costs of nonuniformity. Each organization was asked to provide any information available on the costs of monitoring individual State legislative and regulatory activities, product negotiations with individual States having unique labeling requirements, legal confrontations over individual State requirements, and retrieval, relabeling, and scrapping of products and labels. The companies and trade associations contacted included:

Borden Foods
General Mills
Grocery Manufacturers
  of America
Kellogg Company
Kraft General Foods, Inc.
Land O'Lakes

National Food Processors
  Association
Pepsico-Frito Lay
Procter & Gamble
Quaker Oats Company
RJR Nabisco

Each company and association provided comments to the Committee on condition that the data be compiled and used to represent industry-wide experience. All of the respondents agreed that the costs of these activities are borne by the food manufacturer but that in many cases they are passed on to the consumer as an increment in the price of processed food. None of the companies and associations could provide total dollar costs for the four activities of interest. All concluded, however, that significant continuing costs occur as a result of nonuniformity of Federal and State requirements. Industry incurs these costs in particular in the monitoring of States' activities and product negotiations with States that have unique requirements. Several companies discussed the cost of legal confrontations over individual State requirements and the cost of product retrieval, relabeling, and, at times, scrapping a product and/or its labels. In all cases, examples were cited, but total cost information for all labeling activities concerned with nonuniformity could not be provided.

The Committee recognized that the cost figures provided by the industry were principally anecdotal. However, in the absence of any formalized data, and recognizing the conservative nature of the figures, the Committee concluded that they would serve to adequately illustrate the concerns of industry. The Committee also recognized that nonuniform State requirements could result in significant savings for consumers in such aspects as reduced health costs, while at the same time, resulting in higher food costs. There was no information available to the Committee for evaluation of the costs and benefits to consumers of nonuniform food label requirements.

Monitoring of Individual State Legislative and Regulatory Activities

The magnitude of this activity for a particular firm depends on the types of foods it manufactures. For example, dairy products and dairy substitutes shipped in interstate commerce generally require greater monitoring because this group of foods is especially governed by unique statutes, regulations, and standards that have been established in some States.

The volume of State legislation on labeling—and the concomitant need for monitoring by industry—is reflected in a recent FDA summary of its State legislative monitoring activities. The summary covers 12 major subject areas for the past 2 years. In 1990, the FDA State Program Coordination Branch tracked approximately 3,500 State bills related to food and drugs, of which 109 were concerned with food labeling and 11 were enacted (FDA, 1991a). In 1989, more than 3,000 bills were tracked; 118 related to food labeling, and 18 were enacted (FDA, 1990a).

Most large companies reported having from 1 to 10 employees who monitor State activities at a cost of approximately $80,000 per person. (One large company reported that it also monitors State activities through outside legal counsel at a cost of about $350,000 per year.) Smaller companies frequently employ outside legal or other professional counsel in monitoring, particularly if their food products fall into categories for which some States have unique requirements. One medium-sized manufacturer estimated that it maintains the equivalent of 4 full-time professionally trained people simply to monitor State legislative and regulatory activities, particularly in the dairy products category. A number of companies maintained that many small manufacturers do not have full-time professional people to follow

State activities but instead rely on industry precedents in the labeling of their foods.

FDA lists approximately 20,000 food manufacturers in its inventory of firms that are subject to Federal regulation (FDA, 1990b). If one assumes that, among these firms, only 1,000 of them have an average of one professional person on staff or serving them as outside counsel to monitor State activities, and each of these people is paid a salary plus benefits averaging $80,000, the cost of monitoring for nonuniformity of Federal and State requirements would total approximately $80 million per year. It should be noted that not all of this cost would be focused on State activities related to food labeling requirements. Some of the monitoring activities performed by these individuals would be related to Federal food regulatory activities or Federal and State issues other than labeling of foods. Some of the activities would be expected to continue even if uniformity was established; however, the estimate of 1,000 food processors with professional monitoring capability—and costs—is probably quite conservative, suggesting that the true cost of monitoring is much higher than projected.

Product Negotiations with Individual States Having Unique Labeling Requirements

Negotiations often precede the introduction of a new product in States that have unique requirements for foods in the category into which the new product falls. Frequently, this activity will require as many as three or four meetings involving as many as three or four professional people from the manufacturer's staff and/or the firm's legal counsel. Frequently negotiations are related to foods in the category of dairy products and substitutes, but a number of other negotiations involve the naming of foods that contain artificial flavors and the selection of unique package designs. Some manufacturers report that they cannot sell a new dairy product in a particular State until that State establishes a standard for the new product, which often requires repeated meetings and negotiations involving both corporate personnel and outside legal counsel. The Committee was unable to obtain information on the cost to States of having to carry out such negotiations, because costs are not allocated to specific sections of the law. The total amount is undoubtedly substantial, however, even if measured only in terms of the time spent by State regulators.

In responding to the Committee's questions, some companies commented that negotiations with States having unique requirements impeded the development of new foods. They argued that the uncertainties of State requirements limited the choice of ingredients and thereby delayed the completion of new food formulations. They further noted that if these negotiations are not carried out prior to the introduction of the product, they run the risk that a State with unique requirements may take exception to a product's labeling. When this occurs, product retrieval, relabeling, and legal confrontations can result.

Again, manufacturers could not provide total costs for these negotiations. However, an estimate of $2.5 million is not unreasonable, if one assumes that during the past 3 years, half of all large and medium-sized companies (approximately 500 firms) have averaged one such negotiation at a minimum cost of $5,000 (for travel, personnel, and legal costs).

Legal Confrontations Over Individual State Requirements

Over the years, legal confrontations have generally resulted when manufacturers are confronted with a State's unique requirements for food product names and labeling claims. Such activities can be extremely costly to manufacturers both in the legal and corporate efforts that are expended and the damage done to the reputation of otherwise safe and wholesome foods. One large processor estimates that it spent about $10 million over a relatively short period of time on legal confrontations with a single State. The cost to the State was also undoubtedly significant, considering the time and effort expended by State officials in prosecuting the case. This example is unquestionably one of the most extreme in recent years, but it clearly demonstrates the impact such disagreements can have on the overall cost of food processing. Most companies make every effort to avoid litigation with States; nevertheless, some issues are of such importance to a company that litigation is the only means of resolution. Considering the lack of data in this area, it is not possible to estimate the total costs of such activities to industry.

Product Retrieval, Relabeling, and Scrapping of Product and Labels

These activities generally occur when there has been a breakdown in communication between the State taking action and the company involved. Sometimes the company is not aware of the State's particular requirement and simply distributes the food without recognizing the risk. An example of missed communication occurred in the case of such product names as "chocolate," "chocolate flavored," and "artificially chocolate flavored" foods. The industry has generally followed Federal guidelines in naming these foods; thus, "chocolate" is used in labeling when standardized chocolate is used as the flavor, "chocolate flavored" is used when cocoa is the basic flavor, and "artificially chocolate flavored" is used when the product contains an imitation chocolate flavor. In the past, some States have disagreed with this rationale and insisted that "chocolate" be used only when standardized food chocolate is the basic flavoring; "artificial" or "imitation" chocolate must be used in all other flavor systems, including the use of cocoa. Some States have also taken exception to package size and design, initiating action on the grounds that the product was slack filled or deceptive in design, even though Federal requirements (which may be the minimum) were met.

Retrieval of food products is a difficult task and frequently requires the efforts of sales, manufacturing, and outside personnel. One complicating factor is that product distribution systems often serve multiple States. In those instances, stocks of products in adjoining States, and sometimes ones that are even quite distant from the State in question, must be examined and removed from the system.

Products retrieved from a State can be distributed to other States that do not have such a requirement, but this kind of transfer can only be done on a temporary basis because most distribution systems cannot efficiently separate stocks being sent to individual States. As a result, most companies will relabel their entire product to avoid any further problems in the State with unique requirements. Frequently, large label inventories are on hand when the State files a notice of its action, necessitating the destruction of the old labels when the new ones become available.

Disposal of retrieved products can also be a problem for the food industry. Relabeling previously packaged products is a costly operation because either the old label must be removed and replaced with the approved one or the entire contents must be repackaged and labeled in accordance with a State's requirements. To avoid this expense, firms often find it more expeditious to scrap the retrieved food in a landfill or give it to appropriate charities.

There is no way to estimate the total cost of these actions to the industry, but individual companies have reported on occasion up to as much as $100,000 in product retrieval and scrapping costs and $100,000 in label scrapping costs alone. These costs can be particularly burdensome to small companies that cannot otherwise absorb expenses of this magnitude but must pass them on to consumers in future production.

The Practical Value of Uniform Labeling

In comments to the Committee, industry made it clear that many manufacturers feel that the economic impact of nonuniformity has been part of the cost of food manufacturing in the United States. Industry has known that disparities existed, and generally firms have taken action to avoid confrontations. If a company did run afoul of a unique State requirement, it paid the consequences and took appropriate action to avoid a recurrence. Occasionally, however, situations would arise that pointed up the undesirable costs and administrative problems that are present when great disparities exist.

State regulators may also be uncomfortable with the broad differences between Federal and State requirements that they must enforce. Some of them privately recognize that the differences often stem from laws or regulations that protect home State industries; they may also consider a lack of adequate or clear guidance from Federal agencies to be part of the problem (Corbin, 1991; Sowards, 1991). In either case, in their comments to the Committee, industry representatives showed that they believed that State officials are frequently uncomfortable when they are forced to take a position that appears to be at variance with that of the rest of the country (e.g., States with unique dairy requirements).

The industry's concern over nonuniformity can be even better understood when it is recognized that there are at least 77,600 food labels that are used by some 20,000 food processing firms (FDA, 1990b). A single label printing change incurs an estimated cost of $1,000 to prepare a new single-color label printing plate. Some food manufacturers produce private-label brands for the retail market and other processors; as a result, a single label change may affect all the brands the manufacturer produces. Many foods are also produced in multiple sizes and flavors, and label changes frequently will be required for all of them. The cost of new labels to meet individual State requirements is not insignificant, but it can appear as a subordinate cost when label and product inventories must be scrapped to meet a State's requirements.

States and consumer groups have often suggested that industry should produce multiple labels to meet the requirements of individual States. This approach has been considered many times by food companies, and virtually all have concluded that the distribution system in the United States would be unable to efficiently deliver the properly labeled food to the State(s) having different requirements. Supermarket chains and manufacturers have warehouses that frequently serve multiple States. In practical terms, multiple labels for the same food could not be segregated to ensure that the appropriately labeled food reached its proper destination.

The timing of current efforts to improve uniformity of Federal and State labeling requirements also has implications for U.S. participation in the international marketplace. Europe is now attempting to standardize labeling and other requirements for food products. Through the Codex Alimentarius and other agencies, the United States ultimately will be drawn into this activity. It seems appropriate that the nation resolve its internal labeling differences in preparation for effective participation in the international food trade.

COMMITTEE OBSERVATIONS

The new authority granted to FDA by NLEA will undoubtedly strain its resources at the same time that it affects the authority of States through preemption of their regulations and provisions. State officials and consumer groups have expressed concern over these changes because of their strong belief that implementation of the labeling provisions of FDCA is directly related to the level of enforcement applied by regulators. The Committee believes that the implementation of NLEA should not adversely affect the established cooperative efforts of FDA and the States. The importance of accessible administrative procedures for the exemption petition process and State enforcement of Federal requirements cannot be overemphasized, and FDA must respond to such requests from States in a timely manner.

At the same time, the Committee recognizes that nonuniformity in food labeling has the potential to increase the cost of food to consumers. Any increased cost as a result of nonuniformity is significant, if the interests of consumers are not being served. It is not possible, however, to weigh the costs and benefits of allowing nonuniform State regulations generally or specifically under the six provisions studied in this report. Therefore, the ultimate judgment about consumer benefit may turn out to be largely a matter of preference. Finally, although NLEA assigns responsibilities to FDA that will require the support of the States to fulfill, the responsibility for ensuring that NLEA works goes beyond FDA and the State regulatory agencies. Federal and State legislators and administrators must recognize the importance of food labeling to consumers and provide the resources necessary for meaningful nationwide enforcement activities.

REFERENCES

AFDO (Association of Food and Drug Officials). 1991. Letter to Committee on State Food Labeling, Food and Nutrition Board, Institute of Medicine, Washington, D.C. July 1.

Bryson, C.F. 1991. State Preemption Under Nutrition Labeling and Education Act of 1990. Paper prepared for the Committee on State Food Labeling, Food and Nutrition Board, Institute of Medicine, Washington, D.C. Unpublished.

Burditt, G., Burditt, Bowles, & Radzius, Chartered. 1991. Letter to Burton I. Love, Chair, Food Labeling and Standards Committee, Association of Food and Drug Officials. Feb. 4.

Corbin, L. 1991. Presentation by Leroy Corbin, Pennsylvania Department of Agriculture before the Committee on State Food Labeling, Food and Nutrition Board, Institute of Medicine, May 30.

Crawford, B., Florida Department of Agriculture and Consumer Services. 1991. Letter to Committee on State Food Labeling, Food and Nutrition Board, Institute of Medicine, Washington, D.C. July 5.

CSPI/CNI/CFA/NCL (Center for Science in the Public Interest, Community Nutrition Institute, Consumer Federation of America, and the National Consumers League). 1991. Statement of Sharon Lindan, Assistant Director for Legal Affairs, CSPI, on behalf of CSPI/CNI/CFA/NCL at the Public Meeting of the Committee on State Food Labeling, Food and Nutrition Board, Institute of Medicine, Washington, D.C. May 30.

DHHS (Department of Health and Human Services). 1991. Final Report of the Advisory Committee on the Food and Drug Administration. Washington, D.C.: Government Printing Office.

FDA (Food and Drug Administration). 1990a. Annual Report on State Legislation for the Year 1989. State Program Coordination Branch, Division of Federal–State Relations. Rockville, Md.: FDA.

FDA. 1990b. Food Labeling; Reference Daily Intakes and Daily Reference Values; Mandatory Status of Nutrition Labeling and Nutrient Content Revision; Serving Sizes; Proposed Rules. Fed. Reg. 55:29475–29533; July 19.

FDA. 1991a. Annual Report on State Legislation for the Year 1990. State Program Coordination Branch, Division of Federal-State Relations. Rockville, Md.: FDA.

FDA. 1991b. Food Labeling; General Provisions; Nutrition Labeling; Nutrient Content Claims; Health Claims; Ingredient Labeling; State and Local Requirements; and Exemptions; Proposed Rules. Fed. Reg. 56:60366–60878; Nov. 27.

Gardner, S., and T. Guarino, Grocery Manufacturers of America. 1991. Letter to the Committee on State Food Labeling, Food and Nutrition Board, Institute of Medicine, Washington, D.C. June 19.

Haas, E., Public Voice for Food & Health Policy. 1991. Letter to the Committee on State Food Labeling, Food and Nutrition Board, Institute of Medicine, Washington, D.C. July 10.

Harden, B., Maryland Department of Mental Health and Hygiene. 1991. Letter to the Committee on State Food Labeling, Food and Nutrition Board, Institute of Medicine, Washington, D.C. May 30.

Heffron, E.C., Michigan Department of Agriculture. 1991. Letter to the Committee on State Food Labeling, Food and Nutrition Board, Institute of Medicine, Washington, D.C. July 11.

Lindan, S., Center for Science in the Public Interest. 1991. Letter to the Committee on State Food Labeling, Food and Nutrition Board, Institute of Medicine, Washington, D.C. May 15.

Masso, T., Minnesota Department of Agriculture. 1991. Letter to the Committee on State Food Labeling, Food and Nutrition Board, Institute of Medicine, Washington, D.C. Sept. 10.

McClellan, D., Utah Department of Agriculture. 1991. Letter to the Committee on State Food Labeling, Food and Nutrition Board, Institute of Medicine, Washington, D.C. July 8.

Mitchell, Charles P. 1990. State regulation and federal preemption of food labeling. Food Drug Cosmetic Law J. 45:123–141.

NFPA (National Food Processors Association). 1991. Letter to Dockets Management Branch (HFA-305), Food and Drug Administration, re: Docket 91 N-0038. May 13.

Niles, R., Georgia Department of Agriculture. 1991. Letter to the Committee on State Food Labeling, Food and Nutrition Board, Institute of Medicine, Washington, D.C. June 17.

Rudd, J., Arizona Consumers Council. 1991. Letter to the Committee on State Food Labeling, Food and Nutrition Board, Institute of Medicine, Washington, D.C. July 15.

Sevchik, J., New York Department of Agriculture and Markets. 1991. Letter to the Committee on State Food Labeling, Food and Nutrition Board, Institute of Medicine, Washington, D.C. July 30.

Silverglade, B.A. 1990. Preemption–The Consumer Viewpoint. Food Drug Cosmetic Law J. 45:143–149.

Sowards, R.D., Association of Food and Drug Officials. 1991a. Presentation before the Committee on State Food Labeling, Food and Nutrition Board, Institute of Medicine, Washington, D.C. May 30.

Sowards, R.D., Association of Food and Drug Officials. 1991b. Comments provided to the Committee on State Food Labeling, Food and Nutrition Board, Institute of Medicine, Washington, D.C. July 1.

Thompson, M., Special Counsel, Arnold & Porter. 1991. Letter to G. Burditt, Burditt, Bowles, and Radzius, Chartered. April 17.

U.S. Congress, Senate. 1990. Nutrition Labeling and Education Act of 1990. Congressional Record. S16608–16611. Oct. 24.

Wilms, H., Division of Federal-State Relations, Food and Drug Administration. 1991a. Uniformity of Federal and State enforcement procedures. Presentation before the Committee on State Food Labeling, Food and Nutrition Board, Institute of Medicine, Washington, D.C. May 29.

Wilms, H., Division of Federal-State Relations, Food and Drug Administration. 1991b. Uniformity of Federal and State enforcement procedures. Written comments submitted to the Committee on State Food Labeling, Food and Nutrition Board, Institute of Medicine, Washington, D.C. May 29.

Young, F.E., Food and Drug Administration. 1989. Speech to the American Legislative Exchange Council, Washington, D.C. April 28.

APPENDIXES

A

Provision for the State Food Labeling Study Contained in the Nutrition Labeling and Education Act of 1990

(b) STUDY AND REGULATIONS—

(1) For the purpose of implementing section 403A(a)(3), the Secretary of Health and Human Services shall enter into a contract with a public or nonprofit private entity to conduct a study of—
    (A) State and local laws which require the labeling of food that is of the type required by sections 403(b), 403(d), 403(f), 403(h), 403(i)(1), and 403(k) of the Federal Food, Drug, and Cosmetic Act, and
    (B) the sections of the Federal Food, Drug, and Cosmetic Act referred to in subparagraph (A) and the regulations issued by the Secretary to enforce such sections to determine whether such sections and regulations adequately implement the purposes of such section.
    (2) The contract under paragraph (1) shall provide that the study required by such paragraph shall be completed within 6 months of the date of the enactment of this Act.
    (3)(A) Within 9 months of the date of the enactment of this Act, the Secretary shall publish a proposed list of sections which are adequately being implemented by regulations as determined under paragraph (1)(B) and sections which are not adequately being implemented by regulations as so determined. After publication of the lists, the Secretary shall provide 60 days for comments on such lists.
    (B) Within 24 months of the date of enactment of this Act, the Secretary shall publish a final list of sections which are adequately being

implemented by regulation and a list of sections which are not adequately being implemented by regulations. With respect to a section which is found by the Secretary to be adequately implemented, no State or political subdivision of a State may establish or continue in effect as to any food in interstate commerce any requirement which is not identical to the requirement of such section.

(C) Within 24 months of the date of the enactment of this Act, the Secretary shall publish proposed revisions to the regulations found to be inadequate under subparagraph (B) and within 30 months of such date shall issue final revisions. Upon the effective date of such final revisions, no State or political subdivision may establish or continue in effect any requirement which is not identical to the requirement of the section which had its regulations revised in accordance with the subparagraph.

(D)(i) If the Secretary does not issue a final list in accordance with subparagraph (B) the proposed list issued under subparagraph (A) shall be considered the final list and States and political subdivisions shall be preempted with respect to sections found to be adequate in such proposed list in accordance with subparagraph (B).

(ii) If the Secretary does not issue final revisions of regulations in accordance with subparagraph (C), the proposed revisions issued under such subparagraph shall be considered the final revisions and States and political subdivisions shall be preempted with respect to sections the regulation of which are revised by the proposed revisions.

(E) Subsection (b) of section 403A of the Federal Food, Drug and Cosmetic Act shall apply with respect to the prohibition prescribed by subparagraph (B) and (C).

SOURCE: Nutrition Labeling and Education Act of 1990; Public Law 101-535.

B

Participants at the Public Meeting* Held by the Committee on State Food Labeling, May 30, 1991

RICHARD FRANK, Partner, Olsson, Frank & Weeda, P.C.; representing the Quaker Oats Company and Schreiber Foods, Inc.

SHERWIN GARDNER, Vice President of Science and Technology, Grocery Manufacturers of America

DENNIS R. JOHNSON, Partner, Olsson, Frank & Weeda, P.C.; representing the National Frozen Pizza Institute

SHARON LINDAN, Assistant Director of Legal Affairs, Center for Science in the Public Interest; also representing Community Nutrition Institute, Consumer Federation of America, and National Consumers League

ALLEN MATTHYS, Director, Technical and Regulatory Affairs, National Food Processors Association

DAN SOWARDS, Chair, Food Committee, Association of Food and Drug Officials

MERRILL THOMPSON, Special Counsel, Arnold & Porter; representing Kraft General Foods

FRANCIS WILLIAMS, Executive Director, National Frozen Pizza Institute

*Anyone who asked in advance to speak at the public meeting was given an opportunity to do so.

C

Letter of Request Sent to State and Local Regulators and Consumer Groups by the Committee on State Food Labeling

Dear [State Food Regulator]:

On behalf of the Institute of Medicine's Committee on State Food Labeling, I would like to take this opportunity to thank you for sending the materials that you and your staff provided on your State laws and regulations that are relevant to our study.

As you know, the Committee on State Food Labeling is charged with evaluating the adequacy of Federal regulations addressing six sections related to misbranding in the Food, Drug, and Cosmetic Act (FDCA) as required by the Nutrition Labeling and Education Act of 1990 (NLEA). The Committee is engaged in a six-month study to:

a. assemble a list of all relevant State and local statutes dealing with six misbranding sections of FDCA that will be *preempted* under NLEA;

b. describe the provisions of each State and local statute which pertains to the sections under study and the basis upon which the provisions were developed;

c. assess the extent to which each of the six sections of FDCA are being implemented under current and proposed regulations and evaluate existing data on the impact to public health and nutrition, consumer protection and economics; and

169

d.   make recommendations to FDA on the adequacy of Federal regulations in addressing the six sections of FDCA and identify those State/local statutes that should be considered for Federal adoption.

The Committee on State Food Labeling is seeking to obtain comments on State and local statutes, and their impact and rationale in relationship to the adequacy of Federal regulations for the six sections of the law under study. Those misbranding provisions being examined include:

1.   food under the name of another food [Sec. 403(b)]
2.   container fill and deceptive packaging [Sec. 403(d)]
3.   placement of required information [Sec. 403(f)]
4.   standard of quality and fill [Sec. 403(h)]
5.   common or usual name [Sec. 403(i)(1)]
6.   labeling of artificial flavors, colors, or chemical preservatives [Sec. 403(k)]

In addition to the materials you have sent, the Committee would like to have your comments on the following questions in order to complete our information gathering.

1.   What is your State's perspective on the adequacy of Federal regulations in the six areas that the Committee must address?
2.   What impact do you anticipate preemption of these sections will have on relevant statutes in your State/locality?
3.   Is it important for consumer protection and public health that your State regulation be maintained or adopted as a Federal regulation?
4.   Are there "of the type" statutes in your State of which the Committee should be aware (either in your agency or another state agency charged with administering such statutes)?
5.   Is there case law in your State concerned with any of the six issues that are to be addressed in this study that the Committee should consider?
6.   Are there any other issues that you believe should be brought to the Committee's attention as it deliberates on recommendations to FDA concerning preemption of your State statutes?

The Committee on State Food Labeling would appreciate your answers to any of these questions that are relevant to your State. We need your answers as soon as possible, but no later than July 15, 1991. Please mail your responses to:

Donna V. Porter, Ph.D.
National Academy of Sciences
IOM-FNB 2137-308
2101 Constitution Ave, N.W.
Washington, DC 20418

If you have further questions, please contact the Project Director, Donna Porter [. . .] please leave a message on the answering machine, if she is not available.

The Committee's Vice Chair, Mary Heslin joins me in thanking you in advance for your assistance in answering these questions.

Sincerely yours,

J. Paul Hile
Chair, Committee on
State Food Labeling

cc: State Governor
        Donna V. Porter, Project Director

NOTE: These questions were modified slightly depending upon the recipient of the letter (e.g., state and local regulators, or consumer groups).

D

States Providing Written Response to the Six Questions from the Committee on State Food Labeling

Alabama
Alaska
Arizona
Arkansas
California
Colorado
Connecticut
Delaware
Florida
Georgia
Hawaii
Illinois
Indiana
Iowa
Maine
Maryland
Michigan
Minnesota
Missouri
Montana

Nebraska
Nevada
New Mexico
North Carolina
North Dakota
Oklahoma
Oregon
Pennsylvania
Rhode Island
South Carolina
South Dakota
Tennessee
Texas
Utah
Vermont
Virginia
Washington

Total 37

E

Individuals from States That Provided Information to the Committee on State Food Labeling

Alabama
SHERRY BRADLEY, Division of Food and Lodging Protection, Department of Public Health
BILLY W. KNIGHT, Director, Division of Food and Lodging Protection, Department of Public Health
MARVIN V. TAUNTON, Chief, Food and Drug Inspection, Department of Agriculture

Alaska
KIT BALLENTINE, Acting Director, Division of Environmental Health, Department of Environmental Conservation
ELIZABETH L. SHAW, Assistant Attorney General, Office of the Attorney General

Arizona
STEVEN J. ENGLENDER, Assistant Director, Division of Disease Prevention, Department of Health Services
JOEL RUDD, Vice President, Arizona Consumers Council

Arkansas
SANDRA K. LANCASTER, Program Administrator, Food Protection Services, Division of Sanitarian Services, Department of Health

California
JACK M. SHENEMAN, Food and Drug Scientist, Food and Drug Branch, Department of Health Services

Colorado
SANDY FRAZZINI, Administrative Officer, Consumer Protection Division, Department of Health

Connecticut
KATHLEEN CURRY, Chief, Consumer Affairs Bureau, Department of Consumer Protection
GLORIA SCHAFFER, Commissioner, Department of Consumer Protection

Delaware
FREDERIC L. STIEGLER, Jr., Health Systems Protection, Delaware Health and Social Services, Division of Public Health

Florida
BOB CRAWFORD, Commissioner, Department of Agriculture and Consumer Services
BETSY WOODWARD, Chief, Food Laboratory, Division of Chemistry, Department of Agriculture and Consumer Services

Georgia
RAY NILES, Assistant Director, Consumer Protection Division, Department of Agriculture

Hawaii
MAURICE TAMURA, Chief, Food and Drug Branch, Department of Health

Idaho
DONALD R. BROTHERS, Supervisor, Food Protection Program, Bureau of Preventive Medicine, Division of Health, Department of Health and Welfare

Illinois
ROBERT L. FLENTGE, Chief, Division of Food, Drugs, and Dairies, Department of Public Health
Indiana
GEORGE C. JONES, Administrator, Wholesale Food Protection Program, Division of Wholesale Consumer Affairs, Indiana State Board of Health

Iowa
ARTHUR W. ANDERSON, Division Administrator, Department of Inspections and Appeals

Kansas

JAMES A. PYLES, Administrative Officer, Food and Drug Section, Bureau of Environmental Health Services, Division of Health, Department of Health and Environment

STEPHEN N. PAIGE, Director, Bureau of Environmental Health Services, Division of Health, Department of Health and Environment

Kentucky

JOHN DRAPER, Acting Supervisor, Cabinet for Human Resources, Department for Health Services, Food Branch, Division of Local Health

ROBERT W. CONNATSER, Supervisory Consumer Safety Officer, Investigations Branch, Cincinnati District Office, Department of Health and Human Services, Public Health Service

Louisiana

WILLIAM D. SWILER, Program Manager, Food and Drug Unit, Department of Health and Hospitals

Maine

ERIC J. BRYANT, Assistant Attorney General

Maryland

BETTY HARDEN, Chief, Division of Food Control, Department of Health and Mental Hygiene

Massachusetts

RICHARD D. WASKIEWICZ, Deputy Director, Division of Food and Drugs, Department of Public Health

BETH ALTMAN, Assistant Director, Division of Food and Drugs, Department of Public Health

Michigan

E.C. HEFFRON, Director, Food Division, Department of Agriculture

NEAL FORTIN, Standards Coordinator, Food Division, Department of Agriculture

Minnesota

THOMAS W. MASSO, Director, Food Inspection Division, Department of Agriculture

Mississippi
NORRIS ROBERTSON, Jr., Director, Milk Sanitation Branch, Department
   of Health
CHARLENE BRUCE, Department of Health

Missouri
JOHN NORRIS, Coordinator, Food, Labeling, and Drug Control, Bureau
   of Community Sanitation, Department of Health

Montana
CAL CAMPBELL, Consultant Sanitarian, Food and Consumer Safety
   Bureau, Department of Health and Environmental Sciences

Nebraska
GEORGE H. HANSSEN, Food Division Manager, Department of Agri-
   culture
MARILYN B. HUTCHINSON, Assistant Attorney General

Nevada
JOSEPH L. NEBE, Chief Deputy Food and Drug Commissioner, Depart-
   ment of Human Resources, Health Division, Consumer Health
   Protection Services
ROBERT GRONOWSKI, Director, Division of Plant Industry, Department
   of Agriculture

New Hampshire
JEAN E. BERGMAN, Legal Coordinator, Division of Public Health
   Services

New Jersey
KENNETH KOLANO, Chief, Food and Milk Program, Department of
   Health, Division of Epidemiology and Communicable Disease
   Control

New Mexico
ANTHONY H. SMITH, Environment Department, District I
GARY D. WEST, Department of Agriculture, Division of Standards and
   Consumer Services
EDWARD L. HORST, Health Program Manager, Health and Environment
   Department

New York
DONNELLY C. WHITEHEAD, Senior Inspector, Department of Agriculture and Markets
JAMES L. SEVCHIK, Chief Inspector, Department of Agriculture and Markets

North Carolina
ROBERT L. GORDON, Director, Food and Drug Protection Division, Department of Agriculture
MARTHA DRAKE, President, North Carolina Consumers Council, Inc.
E. BRUCE WILLIAMS, Food Administrator, Food and Drug Protection Division, Department of Agriculture
ALICE LENIHAN, Chief, WIC Section, Department of Environment, Health, and Natural Resources

North Dakota
PERI L. DURA, Director, Department of Health and Consolidated Laboratories

Ohio
PAUL J. SNASHALL, Supervisor, Food, Dairies, and Drugs, Department of Agriculture

Oklahoma
NICK E. SLAYMAKER, Attorney, Department of Health
RICHARD H. BARNES, Director, Food Sanitation Division, Department of Health

Oregon
JAMES A. BLACK, Administrator, Food and Dairy Division, Department of Agriculture

Pennsylvania
LEROY C. CORBIN, Jr., Director, Department of Agriculture, Bureau of Foods and Chemistry
HEATHER S. KOEBERLE, Director, Environmental Health Services, York City Bureau of Health

Puerto Rico
ALFRED C. KING, Director, Department of Health and Human Services, Public Health Service

Rhode Island
RICHARD TURCHETTA, Acting Chief Sanitarian, Division of Food Protection, Department of Health
JENNIFER A. LONGA, Paralegal, Narcotics Unit, Department of the Attorney General

South Carolina
THOMAS W. BROOKS, Assistant Commissioner for Laboratory Services, Department of Agriculture, Consumer Services Division-Laboratory Division

South Dakota
KENNETH SENGER, Director, Division of Public Health, Department of Health

Tennessee
JIMMY HOPPER, Director, Department of Agriculture, Division of Quality and Standards
MARY LOGAN, Food Administrator, Department of Agriculture, Division of Quality and Standards

Texas
JOE K. CREWS, Assistant Attorney General and Chief, Consumer Protection Division, Office of the Attorney General
R.D. SOWARDS, Jr., Chief, Food Branch, Division of Food and Drugs, Department of Health
ELIZABETH M. SCOTT, Paralegal, Consumer Protection Division, Office of the Attorney General
BEVERLY J. WEAVER, Manager, City of Dallas, Food and Commercial Sanitation, Health and Human Services

Utah
DON McCLELLAN, Compliance Officer and Labeling Specialist, Department of Agriculture

Vermont
GEORGE M. DUNSMORE, Commissioner, Department of Agriculture
ALFRED B. BURNS, Sanitarian Supervisor, Agency of Human Services
WILLIAM H. RICE, Assistant Attorney General

Virginia
ARTHUR D. DELL'ARIA, Chief, Bureau of Food Inspection, Department of Agriculture and Consumer Services, Division of Dairy and Foods

Washington
JOHN P. DALY, Assistant Director of Agriculture, Department of Agriculture

West Virginia
Anonymous, Department of Agriculture

Wisconsin
TERRY L. BURKHARDT, Food Labeling Specialist, Food Division, Department of Agriculture, Trade and Consumer Protection

Wyoming
BUD ANDERSON, Food and Drug Compliance Officer, Department of Agriculture

F

State and Local Laws, Regulations, and Other Materials Submitted to the Committee on State Food Labeling

APPENDIX F   State and Local Laws, Regulations, and Other Materials
Submitted to the Committee on State Food Labeling

State/Agencies	Laws	Regulations or Other Materials Submitted
Alabama		
Dept. of Public Health	Food, Drugs, and Cosmetics	General provisions
Dept. of Agriculture and Industries	Food Service Sanitation	Plants and grounds
	Food Processing Establishment Sanitation	Sanitary facilities and controls
		Sanitary operations
		Equipment and procedures
		Production and process controls
		Thermally processed low acid foods packaged in hermetically sealed containers
		Acidified foods
		Cacao products and confectionery
		Smoked and smoke-flavored fish
		Frozen raw breaded shrimp
		Processing and bottling of bottled drinking water
		Permits
		Inspections
		Examination and condemnation of food
		Food processing establishments
		Outside jurisdiction of the health officer
		Review of plans
		Procedure when infection is suspected
		Repealer
Alaska		
Dept. of Environmental Conservation	Agriculture and Animals	Fish inspection
Office of the Attorney General		Labeling requirements
Arkansas		
Dept. of Health	Food, Drug, and Cosmetic Act	No regs.

State/Agencies	Laws	Regulations or Other Materials Submitted
Arizona Dept. of Health Services	Pure Food Control Processed Meat and Meat Product Requirements for Retail Meat Establishments Bottled Water Labeling of Enriched or Fortified Flour, Cereals, and Related Food Products	No regs.
California Dept. of Health Services	Sherman Food, Drug, and Cosmetic Law	No regs.
Colorado Dept. of Health	Pure Food and Drug Law	Labeling of food and consumer commodities
Connecticut Consumer Protection	Pure Food and Drugs Sulfiting Agents Apple Juice, Cider Bottled Water Non-Alcoholic Beverages Labeling, Packaging of Consumer Commodities	Packaging and sale of commodities Proposed regulations for reduced-fat frozen dessert products
Delaware	N.I.P.	N.I.P.
District of Columbia	N.I.P.	N.I.P.
Florida Agriculture and Consumer Services	Milk and Milk Products Law Ice Cream and Frozen Desserts Law Food Processing and Retail Food Sale Citrus Fruit Laws	Milk and milk products rule Ice cream and frozen desserts rules Food processing and retail food sale Shellfish Citrus industry rules
Georgia Dept. of Agriculture	Food Act Vidalia Onion	Packaging and labeling, advertising, and representations in general
Hawaii Food and Drug Branch, Food, Drugs, and Cosmetics	Food, Drug, and Cosmetic Act Bottled Water Intoxicating Liquor Relating to Liquor	Shellfish sanitation

Continued on next page

State/Agencies	Laws	Regulations or Other Materials Submitted
Idaho		
Dept. of Health and Welfare	Food, Drug, and Cosmetic Act	Rules and regulations governing food sanitation standards for food establishments (Unicode)
Illinois		
Public Health	Food, Drug, and Cosmetic Act	Good manufacturing practices for processors of cacao products and confectionery
		Processors of fresh and smoked fish
		Food manufacturing, processing, packing, or holding
		Retail food store sanitation code
		Food service sanitation code
		Grade A pasteurized milk and milk products
		Manufactured dairy products
		Salvage warehouses and stores for foods, alcoholic liquors, drugs, medical devices, and cosmetics
Indiana		
State Board of Health	Uniform Indiana Food, Drug, and Cosmetic Act	N.I.P.
Iowa		
Dept. of Inspections and Appeals	Regulation and Inspection of Foods, Drugs, and Other Articles Adulteration of Foods	N.I.P.
Kansas		
Dept. of Health and Environment, Division of Health	Food, Drug, and Cosmetic Act Honey Law	Food regulations

State/Agencies	Laws	Regulations or Other Materials Submitted
Kentucky Dept. for Health Services	Food, Drug, and Cosmetic Act	Bakery products standard of identity and labeling Food packaging and labeling Labeling guide for food products Shellfish Food and cosmetic salvage regulation
Louisiana Dept. of Health and Hospitals	Food, Drug, and Cosmetic Law	Food, drugs, and cosmetics Bottled water Flour and bread Meat and meat products
Maine Dept. of the Attorney General	Food Law Milk and Milk Products Law Fair Packaging and Labeling Act Products Controlled Act Country of Origin Statute	Labeling fresh produce Frozen dessert products Light/lite dairy products Retail food establishments Food processing and manufacturing Self-service salad/hot food bar retail establishments Mobile vendors Home food manufacturing Fallow deer processing Packaged ice manufacturing and processing Bakeries Food salvage Cider and apple juice plants Maple syrup processing
Maryland Dept. of Health and Mental Hygiene	Misbranded Food Control of Microbial Contamination of Food Exemptions from Labeling Requirements for Foods Subject to Additional Processing, Labeling, or Packing Adulterated Drugs/Devices Standards for Cream Standards for and labeling of Milk Products Grade A Milk Product Dating	Special dietary use rules and regulations

Continued on next page

State/Agencies	Laws	Regulations or Other Materials Submitted
Massachusetts		
Dept. of Public Health	Food, Drugs, and Various Articles	Labeling regulations
Michigan		
Dept. of Agriculture	Food Law of 1968	Hazardous substances
	Comminuted Meat Law	Eggs
	Egg Law	Nonalcoholic beverages
	Weights and Measures Act of 1964	Weights, measures, packaging, and labeling
	Hazardous Substances Act	Consumer pricing and advertising
		False advertising
		Standards of purity for food and drugs
Minnesota		
Dept. of Agriculture	Food Law	Wild rice labeling
		Organic food
Mississippi		
Dept. of Health	Milk and Milk Products Sold at Retail	Bottled water
		Production and sale of milk and milk products
Missouri		
Dept. of Health	Manufacture, Sale, and Distribution of Foods	N.I.P.
Montana		
Dept. of Health	Food, Drug, and Cosmetic Act	Labeling guide for food manufacturers
Nebraska		
Dept. of Agriculture Office of the Attorney General	Pure Food Act	Administrative rules for food
Nevada		
Consumer Health Protection Services	Food, Drugs, and Cosmetics Adulteration Labels, brands	No regs.
New Hampshire		
Dept. of Health and Human Services	N.I.P.	Labeling of raw agricultural products
New Jersey		
Health Dept.	Food, Drug, Cosmetic, and Device Labeling	No regs.

State/Agencies	Laws	Regulations or Other Materials Submitted
New Mexico		
Dept. of Health and Environment	Food Act Flour and Bread Enrichment Act	Retail sale of raw milk Food service and food processor regulations
New York		
Dept. of Agriculture and Markets, Division of Food Inspection Services	Adulteration, Packing, and Branding of Food and Food Products Manufacture, Distribution, and Sale of Maple Syrup and Sugar	Standards of identity and enrichment for cereal flours and related products, milled rice, macaroni and noodle products, and bakery products Labeling of imitation cheese; imitation cheese food and products containing imitation cheese food Fish processing and smoking establishments Manufacture, distribution, and sale of maple syrup and sugar
North Carolina		
Dept. of Agriculture	Food, Drug, and Cosmetic Act	Labeling rules
North Dakota		
Dept. of Health and Consolidated Laboratories	Food, Drug, and Cosmetic Act Beverages Eggs	No regs.
Ohio		
Dept. of Agriculture	Administrative Procedure Act Food, Drug, Cosmetic, and Device Law Administration of the Dairy Trade Practices Law Frozen Dessert Law Dairy Products Law Sanitary Inspection Law Horsemeat Law Vinegar Law Oleomargarine Law and Regulations Foods, Dairies, and Drugs	Authority to promulgate regulations Packaging and labeling regulations and foodstuff ingredient labeling regulations Standards for dairy products Definitions, standards of identity, and requirements for advertising, labeling, quality, and sanitation for imitation milk and nondairy products

Continued on next page

State/Agencies	Laws	Regulations or Other Materials Submitted
Ohio, continued		
Dept. of Agriculture	Laws and Regulations of Maple Products	Milk-O-Tester
	Frozen Food Establishment Law	Regulations for bulk handling of milk from farm to dairy plant
	Ohio Egg Law	Sanitary regulations for
	Candy Law and Regulations Governing Drug Stores, Confectioneries, and Candy FactoriesKosher Food Law	creameries, milk plants, condensaries, and frozen dessert factories
		Standards for raw milk manufacturing purposes
	Soft Drink Bottling Law	and manufactured
	Flour and Bread Enrichment Law	milk plants
		Definitions, standards,
	Sanitary Inspection Law and General Regulations to Promote the Sanitary Condition of Food Establishments	labeling, and tolerances for bread and other bakery products
	Bakery Laws	Sanitary regulations for bakeries
		Meat regulations governing slaughterhouses, poultry dressing plants, and meat markets
		Standards and regulations for salad dressings
		Regulations governing frozen food locker plants and cold storage warehouses
		Naval stores, paint, and linseed oil
		Eggs and egg products
		Standards and regulations for chocolate and cocoa products
		Bottled water regulations
		Sanitary regulations for canneries
		Soft drink bottling regulations
		Macaroni and noodle products
		Corn flour and related products
		Wheat flour and related products
		Bulk food rules of operation

State/Agencies	Laws	Regulations or Other Materials Submitted
Oklahoma Dept. of Health, Food Sanitation Division	N.I.P.	Good manufacturing practice regulations Rules and regulations for the production, processing, and distribution of bottled drinking water
Oregon Food and Dairy Division, Dept. of Agriculture	Food and Other Commodities Food Establishment Standards and Standards for Retail Food Service Activities	Labeling and inspection of meat and meat food products Purity, grades, standards, and labels of dairy products and substitutes Bakeries and bakery products Grades, standards, and labels for agricultural and horticultural products Nonalcoholic beverages Eggs
Pennsylvania Dept. of Agriculture	General Food Law Bakery Law Nonalcoholic Drinks Law Frozen Dessert Law Milk Sanitation Law Milk and Dairy Products Law	Bakery General foods Frozen dessert standards Milk and dairy products general provisions Milk sanitation and standards
Puerto Rico Dept. of Consumer Affairs Dept. of Health Dept. of Agriculture	Food, Drugs, and Cosmetic Act	Labeling prepacked packages Pesticides Poultry and meat marketing Imported bananas and plantains Commercial feed for domestic animals Imported farm products Marketing of sugar Marketing of coffee or coffee products Manufacture and distribution of commercial fertilizer products Marketing of eggs Canning of gandures and their marketing

Continued on next page

State/Agencies	Laws	Regulations or Other Materials Submitted
Rhode Island		
Dept. of the Attorney General	Food, Drug, and Cosmetic Act Truth in Food Disclosure Law Frozen Food Products Farm Milk Holding Tanks Analysis of Milkfat Content in Milk or Milk Product Frozen Dairy Products Meats Poultry Shellfish Packing Houses Pickled Fish Kosher Foods Eggs Milk Sanitation Code Apples Potatoes Fruits and Vegetables Generally Olive Oil Vinegar Nonalcoholic Bottled Beverages, Drinks, and Juices Flour and Bread Corn and Corn Meal Soda and Cream of Tartar Sanitation in Food Establishments	No regs.
South Carolina		
Dept. of Agriculture, Consumer Services Division	Food and Cosmetic Act	Food labeling regulations Packaging and labeling regulations Packing, marketing, and labeling of eggs
South Dakota		
Dept. of Commerce and Regulation	Adulterated and Misbranded Foods	N.I.P.
Tennessee		
Dept. of Agriculture, Division of Markets	Foods, Drugs, and Cosmetics Dairy Law	Packaging and labeling
Texas		
Dept. of Health State Attorney General, Consumer Protection Div.	Food, Drug, and Cosmetic Act	Rules for bottles and vended water

State/Agencies	Laws	Regulations or Other Materials Submitted
Texas (City of Dallas)		
Dept. of Health and Human Services	Misbranded Food	N.I.P.
Utah		
Dept. of Agriculture	Wholesome Food Act	N.I.P.
Governor's Cabinet	Dairy Act	
Vermont		
Dept. of Health	Labeling of Foods, Drugs,	Summary of packaging
Dept. of Agriculture	Cosmetics, and	and labeling regulations
Attorney General	Hazardous Substances	Strawberries
	Product Grades, Standards,	Apples
	and Labeling	Unit pricing
		Fruits and vegetables
		Maple products
		Eggs
		Bait advertising
		Seal of quality regulations: Dairy products, eggs, maple products, potatoes, and sprouts
Virginia		
Dept. of Agriculture and Consumer Services	Virginia Food Laws	N.I.P.
Washington		
Dept. of Agriculture	Food, Drug, and Cosmetic Act	Flour, white bread, and rolls
		Honey
		Ground meat
		Dairies and dairy products
		Fluid milk
		Packaging and labeling regulation
		Perishable packaged food goods – pull dating
West Virginia		
Dept. of Agriculture	Markets	Egg regulations
	Eggs	
	Enrichment of Flour and Bread	
	Imitation Honey	

Continued on next page

State/Agencies	Laws	Regulations or Other Materials Submitted
Wisconsin		
Agriculture, Trade and Consumer Protection	Food Regulations	Retail food establishments Food processing plants Inspection, processing, marketing, and storage of meat and poultry Packaging and labeling Dietary food labeling Label requirements for food products made to resemble a dairy product Grade A milk and milk products: Standards of identity and labeling Reduced fat cheese
Wyoming		
Dept. of Agriculture	None but those of the U.S. FDA	Regulations pertaining to foods, drugs, devices, and cosmetics

NOTES: No regs. = No regs. in addition to State law; N.I.P. = No information provided; FDA = Food and Drug Administration.

G

Areas of Discrepancy Between Federal and State Food Labeling Requirements Identified by States and Consumer and Industry Groups

APPENDIX G   Areas of Discrepancy Between Federal and State Food
Labeling Requirements Identified by States and Consumer and Industry
Groups

State	State Response	Consumer Response	Industry Response
Alabama	N.P.	N.D.I.	Dairy; honey; oysters
Alaska	N.P.	N.D.I.	Fish
Arizona	N.P.	Arizona Consumers Council stated that discrepancies exist between FDCA Sections 403(f), (h), (k) and Arizona law; and requested that FDA adopt Arizona statute (Section 36-906) related to labeling of vegetable fats.	Dairy
Arkansas	N.P.	N.D.I.	Dairy; produce; honey; fish
California	N.P.; however, different bottled water standards. [Personal communication with J. Scheneman, CDHS, who stated that misbranded olive oil is no longer a problem and that the statutory provision is not enforced.]	Bottled water; ice; olive oil; slack fill	Dairy; honey; olive oil
Colorado	N.P.	N.D.I.	Dairy; honey; labeling of bulk food ingredients [FDCA Section 403(k)]
Connecticut	Bottled water; sulfites; apple juice/cider; container fill	Dairy; sulfites; honey	Dairy; honey
Delaware	N.P.	N.D.I.	Dairy; apples (qual./grade); imitation
Florida	Discrepancies between FDCA Sections 403(b), (d), (h), (i) and Florida requirements	Dairy; bottled water; pecans	Dairy; citrus (grade); honey
Georgia	Vidalia onion; also discrepancies between FDCA Sections 403(b), (f), (i)	N.D.I.	Dairy; honey (imitation); Vidalia onion

State	State Response	Consumer Response	Industry Response
Hawaii	Dairy; bottled water; poi; pasta	N.D.I.	Produce (grades); cold-stored foods; bottled water
Idaho	Pending review by attorney general	N.D.I.	Dairy; fruit (grades)
Illinois	N.P.	N.D.I.	Dairy; agric. products (grades)
Indiana	N.P.	N.D.I.	Dairy; produce (grades)
Iowa	N.P.	N.D.I.	Dairy; honey; artificial sweeteners; vinegar; imitation labeling
Kansas	N.P.	N.D.I.	Dairy; produce (grades and qual. stds.); honey
Kentucky	N.P.	N.D.I.	Apples (grade); strawberries (grade)
Louisiana	No response	N.D.I.	Dairy; honey
Maine	Generally no problems except for labeling of cider, MSG added at retail level, and surimi	N.D.I.	Dairy; apples (grade); maple (SI); beverages (colors, flavors, preserv.); cider; surimi; MSG
Maryland	Oysters, free liquor; hen house identity labeling on egg cartons	N.D.I.	Dairy; crab; commodities (stds. of fill)
Massachusetts	No response	Dairy; baking powder; butter/lard; berries (volume); potatoes (grade); canned (prominence); vinegar	Dairy; maple (SI and ingredients); seafood; vinegar; canned food (grade)
Michigan	Diluted fruit beverage standards	N.D.I.	Dairy; apples (grade); buckwheat mixture; composition stds. for red peppers and nutmeg
Minnesota	N.P.	Dairy; label alternatives; wild rice; oysters (fill); smoked fish; fruit syrups jelly; baking powder; salad oil; oranges; prominence for quality and fill; bottled beverages; canned vegetables	Dairy; apples (grade, etc.); honey; wild rice; common name of bulk foods

Continued on next page

State	State Response	Consumer Response	Industry Response
Mississippi	No response	N.D.I.	Dairy; grits (FDCA std.); honey; syrup; catfish
Missouri	N.P. [Law states that regulations must conform as much as practicable to Federal requirements, and be no more stringent; see Missouri State Code, Section 196.050.]	N.D.I.	Dairy; apples (grade); grain mixtures
Montana	N.P.	N.D.I.	Dairy; apples (grade); "Montana farm products"; honey; mustard seed (bug infestations); bottled water
Nebraska	N.P.	N.D.I.	Deceptive packaging
Nevada	N.P.	N.D.I.	Dairy; deceptive packaging of nuts, fruits, and vegetables; potatoes and onions (grades); honey; standard sale units
New Hampshire	No response	N.D.I.	Dairy; apples (grade/qual.); potatoes (grade); "native"; honey; maple (SI, grade, imitation); cider vinegar
New Jersey	No response [NJ has a pending bill on downsizing – Bill 4880, 1991.]	N.D.I.	Dairy; storage of agric. commodities; potatoes (grade)
New Mexico	N.P.	N.D.I.	Dairy; produce; pinon nuts; pecans; honey

State	State Response	Consumer Response	Industry Response
New York	No response	Mellorine; oleo-margarine; horseradish; honey; soaked goods	General authority and standards for milk and dairy products; oleo-margarine; imitation cheese; apples, grapes, lettuce, and potatoes (grades); bulk farm products; honey; ko-sher; maple products; horseradish; baked beans; macaroni (SI); olive oil; vinegar; re-frozen food
North Carolina	N.P.	N.D.I.	Milk (grade/contents); dairy stds. of purity
North Dakota	N.P.	N.D.I.	Non-Federal dairy stds.; imitation dairy labeling; potatoes (grade); organic; flour (weights and measures)
Ohio	No response	N.D.I.	Dairy and frozen des-sert compositional stds.; produce (grades); canned fruit/vegetable labeling (grade/qual.); honey; maple; kosher; soaked canned goods; soft drink "dry" label-ing; bottled water; vinegar; imitation fla-vored soft drinks; mini-mum weight for bread
Oklahoma	N.P.	N.D.I.	Composition stds. for milk; mello-drink; pro-duce (grades); honey; organic; low-alcohol beverages; TVP prod-ucts
Oregon	N.P.	Halibut definition; bac-terial counts for frozen desserts; mellorine; imitation milk and dairy products	SI for milk and frozen desserts; onions, pota-toes, and nuts (grades); bulk agric. products; balloon loaf; flour pro-duct (SI); organic; nonalcoholic beverages stds.; halibut definition

Continued on next page

State	State Response	Consumer Response	Industry Response
Pennsylvania	N.P. [Formaline, metallic copper, honey, and beverage color, etc., labeling provisions repealed in 1909.]	Formaline, etc., in foods; metallic copper; honey; nonalcoholic beverages; colored margarine; benzoic acid-containing products; color labeling; sulfur dioxide use in foods and labeling; lard labeling; oil mixtures labeling; beverage names; nondairy product labeling	Dairy stds.; oleomargarine; produce (grades); honey; chicory with coffee; fruit syrup; vinegar; lard; nonalcoholic beverages; food mixtures; size of type; dairy weights and measures
Rhode Island	N.P.	N.D.I.	Dairy stds.; frozen desserts; exposed surface of fruits; kosher; olive oil mix.; mackerel (grades); cider vinegar
South Carolina	N.P.	N.D.I.	Dairy labeling; frozen desserts; grade stds. for farm products; enriched flour product labeling; rice labeling
South Dakota	N.P.	N.D.I.	Dairy stds.; frozen dessert stds.; potato weight labeling; organic; common or usual names; preservative labeling; water; compound food labeling
Tennessee	N.P.	N.D.I.	Dairy stds.; produce with sulfites (in restaurants); std. weights for margarine
Texas	Generally no problems except for bottled water and alcohol (liquor) in candy	Crabmeat and added chemicals	Produce (grade); bulk agric. products; "self-rising flour"; bread std. sizes; honey; kosher; crabmeat definition; cereal/flour std. weight
Utah	Generally no problems except for bottled water with fruit juice [which should be labeled as a soft drink]; and FDCA Sections 403(f), 403(h), 403(k)	N.D.I.	Dairy stds.; renovated butter; flour/cereal definitions

State	State Response	Consumer Response	Industry Response
Vermont	Generally no problems except for maple syrup SI	Maple syrup SI	Dairy definitions; frozen dessert definitions, qual., and fill; apples (grade); potatoes (grade); maple syrup; organic; irradiated food
Virginia	N.P.	N.D.I.	Dairy stds.; frozen dessert stds.; apples (grade); organic; "Virginia Quality Label"; std. measures for dairy
Washington	No problems in general except for buttered popcorn sold in theaters and fish names	Imitation dairy; halibut names; honey; slack filled products	Dairy; cheese; produce (grades); honey; kosher; organic; halibut; bacon; macaroni; weights and measures for dairy
West Virginia	No response	N.D.I.	Dairy; produce (grades); honey; vinegar; sulfites (restaurants); mixtures; weights and measures for many foods
Wisconsin	No response	N.D.I.	Butter; cheese; imitation dairy; wild rice; weights and measures for many foods
Wyoming	No response	N.D.I.	Dairy; potato (grade/qual. stds.); honey

NOTES:
N.P. = No problems or discrepancies reported.
N.D.I. = No discrepancies identified, or no response received or indicated for a given State.
CDHS = California Department of Health Services.
MSG = monosodium glutamate.
SI = standard of identity.
FDCA = Federal Food, Drug, and Cosmetic Act of 1938, as amended.
TVP = textured vegetable protein.

H

State Food Labeling Requirements and Relationship to the Misbranding Provisions of Section 403 of the Federal Food, Drug, and Cosmetic Act

APPENDIX H State Food Labeling Requirements and Relationship to Misbranding Provisions of Section 403 of the Federal Food, Drug, and Cosmetic Act of 1938, as amended

Food or Commodity	States with Law/Regulation	Description	Federal Requirement	Related FDCA Section 403					
				b	d	f	h	i	k
Bottled water	Arizona; R9-8-204 (regs.) California; §26591 to 94 Connecticut; §21a-150 Delaware; §4315 Florida; 500.455 (regs.) Hawaii; §328D-6 Louisiana; §608(12) and 49:2.1110 (regs.) Maine; Title 36, §1572 Maryland; §21-336 Mississippi; §15.18 (regs.) Montana; §50-31-236 New Jersey; §24:12-9 North Dakota; §19-08-02 Ohio; Title 9, §913.24 Oklahoma; §1-917 Texas; §229.81 to 88	Define standards of quality for bottled waters and define names of waters by source	Standard of quality; 21 CFR §103.35 Processing and bottling of bottled drinking water; 21 CFR Part 129	x	x	x	x	x	x
Halibut	Alaska; §17.20.045 Massachusetts; §194B Oregon; §616.217 Washington; §69.04.315		21 CFR §102.57; Acceptable names are *Hippoglossus hippoglossus* and *Hippoglossus stenolepsis*	x			x		

205

	Establishes standard of identity, standard of quality, grades, and additional labeling requirements.	None; grading under USDA
Honey	Alabama; §2-11-121 and 122	
	Arkansas; §20-57-402	
	California; §29401 to 421; §29448; §29471 to 474; §29501 to 504; §29531; §29581 to 587; §29611 to 620; §29641 to 644; §29671 to 675, §29677	x
	Colorado; §35-25-102, §109	
	Connecticut; §22-181a	
	Florida; §582.02; §586.03; §586.051	x
	Georgia; §26-2-233	
	Iowa; §198.14; §190.1(67)	x
	Kansas; §65-681	x
	Louisiana; §608.1	
	Minnesota; $31.74	
	Mississippi; §75-29-601	
	Nevada; §583.355	
	New Hampshire; §429:22, §429:23	
	New Mexico; §25-9-263	
	New Jersey; §205 and §206	
	New York; §206	
	Ohio; §3715.01, §3715.38	
	Oklahoma; Title 78, §81	

Continued on next page

APPENDIX H—Continued

Food or Commodity	States with Law/Regulation	Description	Federal Requirement	Related FDCA Section 403					
				b	d	f	h	i	k
Honey, continued	Washington; §69.28.020 to 390; §69.28.030; §69.28.400 West Virginia; §19-20-1 and §19-20-2 Wyoming; §11-8-102								
Maple syrup	Maine; Title 7, §891 to 4 Massachusetts; §36C New Hampshire; §429:13 and 14 New York; §203 to 204 Ohio; §3715.24 to 26 Vermont; Title 6, §481, §492, §293	Establishes standard of identity, grades, and additional labeling requirements.	21 CFR §168.140, Standard of identity	x		x	x	x	x
Oysters	Florida; §5E-6.010(8)(d) (regs.) Maryland; 10.15.08.02 (regs.) Minnesota; §1545.2670 (regs.) New York; Art. 17, §212	Establishes levels of "free liquor" allowed in canned oysters; Florida allows 15 percent by volume; Maryland allows 5 percent by volume; Minnesota restricts drained weight to no less than 59%; New York allows 10 percent by volume.	21 CFR §161.3; Declaration of quantity of contents on labels of canned oysters 21 CFR §161.130 to 140; quality and fill standards for 9 varieties of oysters 21 CFR §161.45; canned oysters; drained weight	x		x	x		

Product	State citation	Federal standard		
Olive oil and vegetable oil mixtures	California; §28475 to 78; §28480 to 82; §28484 to 86 (olive oil) Minnesota; §1550.0620 (regs.) (veg. oil mix.) New York; §2-4a (olive oil) Pennsylvania; Title 7, §47.3 (veg. oil mix.) Rhode Island; §21-21-1; §21-21-2; §21-21-6 (olive oil)	None	x	x x
Pecans	Florida; §5E-6.007 (regs.) Georgia; New Mexico; §76-16-1 to 9	None; grading under USDA	x	x x
Surimi	Maine; Title 12, §6111-6112 Maryland; §21-302(1); §21-329 Texas (crab labeling); §241.23(e) (regs.), requires labeling of any added chemical and type of meat (i.e., lump, claw, etc.)	None	x	x

Continued on next page

APPENDIX H—Continued

Food or Commodity	States with Law/Regulation	Description	Federal Requirement	Related FDCA Section 403					
				b	d	f	h	i	k
Vinegar	Connecticut; §21a-146 to 148 Iowa; §190.8; §191.8 Maine; §543-A Massachusetts; §170 and 171 Michigan; §289.552 to 558 New Hampshire; §146:14 New York; §207, §208 Ohio; §3715.28 to 33 Pennsylvania; §921 to 924 Rhode Island; §21-22-1 to 3 West Virginia §19-22-1, 5, 6		None	x		x	x	x	x
Wild rice	Minnesota; §30.49 Wisconsin; §97.57		None	x		x	x		

Free liquor = That liquid portion of the contents of a container that passes through a pervious straining device when the contents (oyster meats) of the container are drained.

I

Case Study: Requirements for Labeling Bottled Water

In the course of its deliberations, the Committee identified a number of instances in which individual States acted in the absence of a Federal regulation. One of the best examples of this practice concerns bottled water. The Committee prepared the following case study of bottled water to examine the type of problems that some States believe to have existed and to explore their regulatory response.

In the past several years, the regulation of bottled water by the Food and Drug Administration (FDA) has been seen by some as an unfortunate paradigm of the effects of deregulation.[1] For its part, FDA has candidly stated that it does not believe that bottled water poses a risk to the public health and so has not devoted substantial resources to its regulation. That decision apparently has not been shared by 23 States, which have adopted statutes or regulations governing the quality or labeling of bottled water. The recent worldwide recall of Perrier mineral water following benzene contamination was seen by some as both proof of FDA's ineffective regulation (the problem was originally discovered in North Carolina) and the industry's inability to police itself. Hearings conducted by the House Committee on Energy and Commerce's Subcommittee on Oversight and Investigations criticized FDA for its regulation of bottled water (U.S. Congress, 1990; U.S. Congress, 1991), following a U.S. General Accounting Office (GAO) report (GAO, 1991) that took the same position.

The regulation of bottled water requires the consideration of two provisions of the Federal Food, Drug, and Cosmetic Act of 1938, as amended (FDCA), that Congress has directed (through the Nutrition Labeling and Education Act of 1990; NLEA) be studied before preemption decisions can be made. The requirements were that a food not subject to a standard of identity bear a common or usual name [FDCA Section

209

403(i)(1)], and the requirement that a food meet any applicable standard of quality or disclose on its label that it does not [FDCA Section 403(h)(1)].

In examining FDA's regulation of bottled water, several ambiguities arose. State standards of identity are preempted if they are not identical to corresponding Federal standards. Similarly, State common or usual name regulations are preempted if it is determined that FDA is adequately implementing the common or usual name requirement of FDCA. But does NLEA permit a State to adopt a standard of identity for a product for which no Federal standard exists? The superficial answer would appear to be yes, since NLEA and the regulations proposed to date do not specifically prohibit a State from doing so. Yet the preemption provision applicable to the common or usual name requirement prohibits "any requirement for the labeling of a food of the type required" by FDCA Section 403(i)(1). It is unclear, however, whether (1) FDA must have established a specific common or usual name for bottled water, or (2) the general provisions of FDCA Section 403(i)(1) and its implementing regulations are sufficient for preemption of any such State requirements. If it is found that FDA is adequately implementing the common or usual name requirement of the statute under either circumstance, and thus preempting this area of State requirements, the question still remains as to whether a State can name a food by issuing a standard of identity.

Another issue surrounds the peculiarities of the bottled water quality standard. Bottled water is the only food for which FDA has adopted a standard of quality in the absence of a standard of identity. Quality standards usually do not deal with issues of food safety, and State regulation of food safety is not preempted by NLEA. Therefore, ambiguity also surrounds the question of whether States can regulate the safety of bottled water in a regulation that is called a quality standard, or whether they can regulate bottled water by calling the regulation one of food safety when in fact it covers the same ground as the FDA quality standard.

Although these problems ultimately must be faced and resolved by FDA, their resolution is viewed as beyond the scope of this case study. As discussed in Chapter 4, the Committee has decided to leave to FDA the decision of whether a State law or regulation is a standard of identity or a common or usual name regulation, and determination of the consequences that flow from that decision.

FDA ADOPTION OF STANDARD OF QUALITY AND GOOD MANUFACTURING PRACTICE REGULATIONS

FDCA Section 401(a) [21 USC §341(a)] authorizes FDA to establish for any food definitions and standards of identity, reasonable standards of quality, and reasonable standards of fill of container. A food that is subject to a quality standard is misbranded if it does not conform to that standard or does not declare on its label that it does not conform [FDCA Section 403(h)(1)]. Until the passage of NLEA, the adoption or amendment of quality standards for all products required the use of formal rulemaking under FDCA Section 701(e).[2]

Exercising its authority under FDCA Section 401, FDA established quality standards for bottled water in 1973. In proposing the standard, the agency explained that "[b]ottled water is increasingly being used as a source of drinking water. . . . The consumer expects bottled water to meet the minimum criteria established for public drinking water supplies" (FDA, 1973a; p. 1019).

The quality standards were based on the 1962 Public Health Service standards for public drinking water supplies. FDA noted then that the recently created Environmental Protection Agency (EPA) had assumed the responsibility for establishing drinking water standards and that FDA intended to revise the bottled water standards to keep them compatible with EPA drinking water standards.

FDA received 33 comments on the proposed standards. These comments raised most of the issues about bottled water that continue to be of concern today. One comment suggested that FDA adopt more stringent standards than those adopted by EPA because many consumers assume that bottled water is of a higher quality than tap water. FDA replied:

> Although some consumers may assume, and some promotion of bottled water may encourage, the assumption that bottled water is of a higher quality than tap water, there is no Federal requirement to this effect. The quality of tap water and bottled water can vary widely due to the source itself . . . as well as to treatments these waters may receive during processing. Because of these source and treatment variables there is no basis for assuming that bottled water is of a higher quality than municipal tap water (FDA, 1973b; p. 32558).

Several comments also suggested that bottled mineral water be subject to the quality standard. FDA concluded that mineral water was "inherently different" from bottled water and that a separate quality standard would be developed. Optimistically, the agency stated that the lack of a quality standard for mineral water would be a "temporary situation" (FDA, 1973b; pp. 32558-32559).

Several State health agencies objected to the proposal because it did not provide for the safety of bottled water. FDA replied that "if bottled water contains any substance at a level injurious to health, it will be deemed to be adulterated and appropriate regulatory action will be taken, whether or not it meets the standard of quality" (FDA, 1973b; p. 32559).

As noted earlier, FDA departed from its usual procedure when it first proposed a standard of quality for bottled water without at the same time proposing a standard of identity. The agency's initial *Federal Register* notice did not explain the rationale for this decision, but several commenters urged FDA to regulate the use of such terms as "spring," "well," and "distilled water." FDA declined and stated:

> [T]here is no need for a requirement that the source or treatment of the water be declared on the label of bottled water. Bottled drinking water can be produced from various sources of water, and various types of treatment of the water can be used in manufacturing bottled water of an acceptable quality. If the manufacturer decides to provide information in the labeling or in advertising relating to bottled water, stating or implying that it is the product of a specific source of water or that the water has been treated in a specific manner, such information must be truthful, factual, and not misleading in any respect. Sec. 403(a) of the act provides that a food shall be deemed to be misbranded if its labeling is false or misleading in any particular. The Commissioner concludes that this statutory authority is sufficient to provide for regulatory action in instances where false or misleading statements concerning the source or treatment of bottled water are made and that specific statements to this effect in the standard are unnecessary (FDA, 1973b; p. 32561).

In addition to citing the general prohibition against false and misleading label claims in FDCA Section 403(a), FDA also could have relied on FDCA Section 403(i), which deems a food misbranded unless it bears its common or usual name. If the source of a particular bottled water was a municipal water supply but the water was labeled as "spring water," it would not only be labeled in a false or misleading manner but would also be misbranded for failing to bear its common or usual name. Although objections to the final rule were filed, FDA concluded that they did not justify changing the regulation or conducting a hearing, and the quality standard became effective on June 19, 1975 (FDA, 1975).

In 1974, passage of the Safe Drinking Water Act codified the division of labor for regulating water between FDA and EPA. In addition to directing EPA to promulgate national primary drinking water standards, the Safe Drinking Water Act also added Section 410 to FDCA. Section 410 directs FDA to consult with EPA whenever the latter issues interim or revised national primary drinking water standards and, within 180 days of EPA's promulgation, either amend the bottled water standard or explain its rationale for not doing so in the *Federal Register*. From 1975 to 1979, FDA met or came close to meeting the 180-day time limit. Since then, however, FDA has not even come close to meeting the statutory deadline for acting on EPA actions.

In 1975, FDA adopted Good Manufacturing Practice (GMP) regulations for bottled water, including bottled mineral water (21 CFR §129.1 *et seq.*). Among other things, these regulations specify the kinds of facilities that must be used and the process controls that are required to ensure a safe product. The regulation also requires that "product water" (i.e., the water that is to be bottled) come from an approved source. "Approved source" is defined as a source of water and the water itself "that has been inspected and the water sampled, analyzed, and found to be of a safe and sanitary quality according to applicable laws and regulations of State and local government agencies having jurisdiction" [21 CFR §129.3(a)]. The regulation also requires that bottled water manufacturers test source water (from other than a public water system) and bottled water as often as necessary but including at least weekly for microbiological contamination and at least yearly for chemical contamination. Testing of source water "shall be consistent with the minimum requirements set forth in [the bottled water quality standard]" [21 CFR §129.35(a)(3)(ii)].

On January 29, 1988, the International Bottled Water Association (IBWA) filed a citizen petition with FDA seeking the amendment of the bottled water quality standards to define the various kinds of bottled water, including mineral water. IBWA also sought amendment of the bottled water GMPs to require source testing and mandatory annual testing by all producers.

CONGRESSIONAL SCRUTINY

The Subcommittee on Oversight and Investigations of the House Committee on Energy and Commerce held a hearing on FDA oversight of bottled water on April 10, 1991. In a memorandum dated April 9 to members of the Subcommittee on Oversight and Investigations outlining the expected testimony, the chairman, John D. Dingell (D-Mich.), said that testimony would show that

> FDA has, in three major ways, abdicated its responsibility to regulate the product: by failing to promptly adopt quality standards, as required by statute; by failing to define bottled water products, despite an 18-year old pledge to do so; and by failing to consider the bottled water industry's proposal to adopt a regulatory model code to assure consumer confidence (Dingell, 1991).

The fundamental difference between the way FDA has traditionally viewed bottled water and the way the subcommittee and perhaps consumers now view the product was evidenced by the following statement by Chairman Dingell:

> Finally, this hearing will address whether consumers can be confident that what they are purchasing is pristine, pure water, possessing unique characteristics that make it

inherently superior to tap water by virtue of its source and its physical properties (Dingell, 1991).

From FDA's point of view, however, it had never purported to regulate bottled water as a product with "unique characteristics that make it inherently superior to tap water." To the contrary, FDA had rejected such an implication in 1973 when it adopted the quality standard for bottled water. It stated then that there is no Federal requirement that bottled water be of higher quality than tap water and "there is no basis for assuming that bottled water is of a higher quality than municipal tap water" (FDA, 1973b). Thus, the subcommittee's criticism seemed largely based on FDA's failure to regulate bottled water in the way the subcommittee now believes it should be regulated, rather than in the way FDA had consistently maintained it would be regulated.

The subcommittee's criticism of FDA also included what appeared to be an unfair assertion that there were 22 recalls of bottled water "for reasons ranging from the detection of mold to contamination by kerosene" (Dingell, 1991). An examination of these recalls shows that the actual situation was not nearly so dire. Five of the 22 were of one product—the benzene-contaminated Perrier mineral water, which was available in unflavored form and in four flavors. These cases were Class II recalls. Similarly, six Class III recalls (the lowest level of regulatory action) concerned mold and yeast contamination of six flavors of the same bottled water product. These products were sweetened, thus making them flavored soda waters rather than bottled waters. Although they were arguably misbranded for failing to state their common or usual name, they were not subject to the bottled water quality standard and should not have been counted as such. Two other manufacturers recalled five products. The subcommittee's list also included a recall of club soda even though club soda is not traditionally considered a bottled water nor is it subject to the bottled water quality standard. A Class I recall of isopropyl alcohol was listed as involving bottled water because it was erroneously labeled as distilled water. This case was a drug recall, not a recall of bottled water (Dingell, 1991). When all of these factors are taken into account, it appears that bottled water recalls were instituted by only seven manufacturers in 1990, an unexceptional record for an industry with more than 450 producers. For the purpose of this study, only six recalls involved actual or potential misbranding charges.

FDA's failure to adopt the industry's requested regulatory scheme does not necessarily mean that the agency was in error. Industry rarely seeks Federal regulation unless it perceives some economic benefit in doing so. In a letter to an association member, the IBWA president stated that "once we have succeeded in establishing federal regulation of our industry through the FDA, we will be in a position to make the strongest public statement possible that we are the most regulated beverage sold in the United States" (Dingell, 1991, attachment G). While being able to make that statement might be helpful for marketing purposes, Americans consume far more colas and soda waters annually, and these beverages are subject to neither the bottled water quality standard nor the bottled water GMPs. They are consumed without health hazard and not regulated at the level of oversight that the bottled water industry is seeking, apparently for marketing purposes.

A GAO report on FDA's regulation of bottled water, prepared at the request of the subcommittee, took FDA to task for failing to observe the time limits set by Congress for adopting EPA's primary drinking water standards (GAO, 1991). GAO also criticized FDA for inspecting bottled water plants only on the average of every 5-3/4 years, failing to require bottlers to use certified laboratories or to report results to FDA (authority that the agency claims it does not have), and failing to define terms frequently found on bottled water labels, such as "spring," "pure," and other quality or source claims. GAO recommended that FDA seek legislation authorizing it to use certified laboratories to test water and to report those results to the agency. It also suggested that Congress might wish to amend FDCA Section 410 to automatically adopt EPA's standards, unless FDA acts.

The GAO report also suggested that the bottled water industry is causing considerable potential health hazards to the public. However, FDA believes that the evidence supports its view that, by and large, the bottled water supply in this country is safe and adequately labeled and simply does not deserve a higher level of regulatory scrutiny.

Fred Shank, director of FDA's Center for Food Safety and Applied Nutrition, gave candid testimony to the subcommittee about the way FDA uses its limited resources to police the U.S. food supply. Dr. Shank (1991) stated unequivocally that

. . . we have no reason to question the safety of bottled water. Based on our experience, FDA considers bottled water to have a low potential for contamination or for causing sickness. . . (p. 1).

Bottled water establishments are included under the general food safety program. In this program bottled water plants generally are assigned low priority for inspection. FDA bases its priorities on factors such as the potential for public health problems and the violation rate of the industry. When compared to products such as low acid canned foods and products where *Listeria* or *Salmonella* have a significant potential to develop, bottled water products must take a back seat. Our experience over the years . . . has not shown that there is a significant problem with bottled water products. . . (p. 12).

[W]e believe bottled water is a safe product. As an industry, bottled water has fewer compliance problems than most other food industries. That is why FDA classifies bottled water as a low risk product. Even the compliance problems the bottled water industry has with FDA have not been of a type that can be classified as a hazard (p. 20).

Notwithstanding this vigorous defense of FDA's actions, it is not surprising that the congressional attention has caused FDA to rethink some of its positions. The subcommittee was told that the agency was reconsidering the coverage of the bottled water standards to include mineral water and the bottled water component in flavored beverage products fabricated from bottled water ingredients. It is also considering a new quality standard requiring the water component of seltzer, tonic water, colas, and similar products to meet quality standards based on EPA's primary drinking water standards. The agency has not spoken to the need for standards of identity or common or usual names.

STATE ACTIONS

A total of 23 States have expressed their dissatisfaction with FDA's regulation of bottled water by adopting laws or regulations to provide additional controls. Although these State laws vary, in general, they address two basic issues: the nomenclature of various types of bottled waters and the purity of the products. (These laws and regulations are summarized in Appendix H.) Many States have adopted the Association of Food and Drug Officials' (AFDO) model bottled water regulation, or some variation of it (AFDO, 1984). The AFDO model regulation contains definitions for the following waters: artesian well, bottled, demineralized, drinking, light mineral, mineral, mineralized, natural, purified, spring, and well. The model regulation requires that all bottled waters bear one of the defined names and that artificially carbonated waters disclose the addition of carbonation. It also requires compliance with the FDA standard of quality, the bottled water GMPs, and source water and finished product sampling (21 CFR Part 129).

In communications to the Committee, a number of States expressed discontent with FDA's inaction in the alleged face of false and misleading labeling claims for bottled water products. Even a cursory examination of supermarket shelves confirms that there are a number of products that could be the subject of FDA enforcement action, based on their labeling. Although the recent growth of the bottled water industry has made the public and regulators more aware of potentially false and misleading labeling, it can be argued that FDA's prioritization of its enforcement resources is sound. In any event, the Committee has determined that whether FDA actually enforces particular statutory provisions is beyond the scope of its inquiry.

ASSESSMENT OF ADEQUACY AND CONCLUSIONS

Much of the recent controversy, and many of the States' regulatory initiatives, have focused on the safety of bottled water. Although of great importance, this issue falls outside of the scope of NLEA and, therefore, this study. On the other hand, the same States that have expressed concern over Federal quality standards have also believed it necessary to establish nomenclature requirements. Some States and consumer groups believe that the opportunity for public confusion has increased by virtue of the increased number of products in the market and the increasingly aggressive claims made for these products.

In 1973, FDA believed it was evident that bottled water was not any better or purer than tap water. That conclusion may still be factually valid, but the Committee questions whether that view is held by consumers after years of exposure to advertising claims of superiority for bottled and mineral water. As mentioned above, the fact that nearly half the States have established definitions for the different types of bottled and mineral waters on the market is evidence that there is a perception that FDA's efforts here have not been adequate. Although the general misbranding provisions of FDCA could have been used by FDA to prosecute many of the perceived offenders, it is clear that the States believed that the existence of definitions in the form of standards or common or usual names would make their enforcement job easier. Based on the Committee's working principles, it can be concluded that the State laws and regulations that define and/or standardize the names of the various kinds of bottled and mineral waters are appropriately candidates for Federal adoption.

NOTES

1. FDA considers "bottled water" to be "water that is sealed in bottles or other containers and intended for human consumption. Bottled water does not include mineral water or any type of soft drink commonly known as soda water, which is made by adsorbing carbon dioxide in potable water" [21 CFR §103.35(a)]. Most State laws dealing with bottled water, as well as the Association of Food and Drug Officials' model bottled water regulation, include mineral water within their ambit. Unless the context dictates otherwise, this paper includes mineral water within the term "bottled water."
2. NLEA Section 8 amends FDCA to permit the issuance and amendment of standards of identity, quality, and fill of container for food products other than dairy products and maple syrup by notice-and-comment rulemaking under FDCA Section 701(a).

REFERENCES

AFDO (Association of Food and Drug Officials). 1984. AFDO Model Bottled Water Code, adopted 1984. York, Pa.: AFDO.

Dingell, J.D. 1991. Memorandum to members of the Subcommittee on Oversight and Investigations, House Committee on Energy and Commerce, U.S. Congress. April 9.

FDA (Food and Drug Administration). 1973a. Bottled Water; Proposed Quality Standards. Fed. Reg. 38:1019–1020; Jan. 8.

FDA (Food and Drug Administration). 1973b. Bottled Water; Quality Standards; Addition of Flouride and Current Good Manufacturing Practice Regulations; Final Rule. Fed. Reg. 38: 32557–32565; Nov. 26.

FDA (Food and Drug Administration). 1975. Quality Standards for Bottled Water; Final Rule. Fed. Reg. 40:21932–21934; May 20.

GAO (U.S. General Accounting Office). 1991. Stronger FDA Standards and Oversight Needed for Bottled Water. GAO, Washington, D.C.

Shank, F.R. 1991. Testimony of Fred R. Shank, Director, Center for Food Safety and Applied Nutrition, Food and Drug Administration, before the Subcommittee on Oversight and Investigations, House Committee on Energy and Commerce, U.S. Congress. April 10.

U.S. Congress, House. 1990. Proceedings of the Bottled Water Workshop, September 13-14, 1990: A report for the Subcommittee on Oversight and Investigations, Committee on Energy and Commerce. Committee print 101-X. Washington, D.C.

U.S. Congress, House. 1991. Bottled Water Regulation. Hearing before the Subcommittee on Oversight and Investigations, Committee on Energy and Commerce. Transcript 102-36. Washington, D.C.

J

Biographical Sketches of Committee Members and Staff

J. PAUL HILE, Chairman, is President of and a Senior Consultant with Phoenix Regulatory Associates, Ltd. From October 1986 to April 1991, he was Director of the Regulatory Affairs Division, Hazelton Corporation. From 1958 to 1986, Paul worked for the Food and Drug Administration in several positions, serving as Associate Commissioner for Regulatory Affairs from 1976 to 1986. Paul is the recipient of many honors from the Food and Drug Administration and the Public Health Service, and is the Editor-in-Chief of *Regulatory Affairs*. He is a member of the Regula-tory Affairs Professionals Society, Institute of Food Technologists, Association of Food and Drug Officials, and Association of Official Analytical Chemists. He holds a B.S. in agriculture from Colorado State University.

MARY HESLIN, Vice Chairman, is Principal Officer of Heslin Consulting and was formerly Commissioner of Consumer Protection for the State of Connecticut from 1975 to 1991. Mary has also served as Deputy Mayor of the City of Hartford and a member of the Hartford City Council. She is a member of the Executive Board of Women Executives in State Government and is past president of the Association of Food and Drug Officials and the National Association of Consumer Agency Administrators. She has received numerous awards, most recently the 1991 Harvey Wiley Award, from the Association of Food and Drug Officials, and has published extensively on consumer protection issues. She holds a B.A. in English from the University of Connecticut and an M.A. in history from Trinity College.

SANDRA O. ARCHIBALD is Assistant Professor of Agricultural Economics at the Food Research Institute, Stanford University. Dr. Archibald is on the board of the Morrison Institute for Population and Resources at Stanford and was previously Economic Director for the Rockefeller Commission for Critical Choices. She has served as a consultant to the National Research Council's Board on Agriculture, the Environmental Protection Agency, and the Department of Interior; she has also advised government agencies on food safety and environmental policy. Sandra has published extensively on agriculture, food safety, and toxicology issues. She holds B.A. and M.A. degrees in public policy from the University of California at Berkeley and M.S. and Ph.D. degrees in agricultural economics from the University of California at Davis.

MARSHA N. COHEN is Professor of Law at Hastings College of the Law, University of California, San Francisco, where she has taught since 1976. Ms. Cohen has served as Staff Attorney and Consultant to Consumers Union of United States, Inc. She was a member of the Health, Education and Welfare Secretary's Review Panel on New Drug Regulation, and has served as Vice President and President of the California State Board of Pharmacy. Marsha holds a B.A. from Smith College and a J.D. from Harvard Law School.

JOHN W. ERDMAN, Jr., is Professor of Food Science and Professor of Nutrition in Internal Medicine at the University of Illinois at Urbana, where he has been on the faculty since 1975. Dr. Erdman is currently Director of the Division of Nutritional Sciences at Illinois. John has served on the editorial boards of a number of food science and nutrition journals, including the *Journal of Nutrition*, for which he is currently Associate Editor. He has received numerous awards and honors. John currently serves on the Institute of Medicine's Food and Nutrition Board and the Committee on Opportunities in the Nutrition and Food Sciences; he is also a member of the Subcommittee on Bioavailability of Nutrients of the Committee on Animal Nutrition of the National Research Council's Board on Agriculture. He holds B.S., M.S., M.Phil., and Ph.D. degrees in food science from Rutgers University.

JESSE F. GREGORY III is Professor and Acting Chair of the Food Science and Human Nutrition Department at the University of Florida, where he has been on the faculty since 1977. He is involved in teaching and research concerning food chemistry, food analysis, and the nutritional quality of foods. His research deals mainly with chemical, analytical, and nutritional aspects of vitamin B_6 and folic acid, with current emphasis on improving our understanding of the bioavailability of these vitamins. He has published extensively in the fields of food science and nutrition. Dr. Gregory has received several awards for research including the 1983 Samuel Cate Prescott Award for Research from the Institute of Food Technologists. He serves on the Editorial Boards of *Nutrition Reviews* and the *Journal of Nutrition*. He holds B.S. and M.S. degrees in food science from Cornell University and a Ph.D. in food science and nutrition from Michigan State University.

TIMOTHY M. HAMMONDS is Senior Vice President of the Food Marketing Institute (FMI) in Washington, D.C., where he is responsible for FMI's research and education programs—pharmacy services, international, and industry relations. He also serves as Co-editor of the professional journal *Agribusiness*. Prior to joining FMI, Dr. Hammonds was Vice President for Research for the Super Market Institute in Chicago and visiting staff economist for the National Association of Food Chains in Washington, D.C. He previously served on the faculty of the Department of Agricultural Economics at Oregon State University. Tim holds a B.S., an M.B.A., and a Ph.D. degree in agricultural economics from Cornell University.

ALVIN J. LORMAN is a partner in the law firm of Akin, Gump, Hauer & Feld in Washington, D.C., practicing in all areas of food and drug law. He has been a Partner and Of Counsel to several Washington law firms and was a Law Clerk for Judge Leonard Braman of the Superior Court of the District of Columbia. Mr. Lorman was the author of *Food Standards and the Quest for Healthier Foods*, a commissioned paper for the Food and Nutrition Board/Institute of Medicine report, *Nutrition Labeling: Issues and Directions for the 1990s*. He holds a B.A. from Long Island University, an M.A. from Ohio State University, and a J.D. from the University of Virginia School of Law, where he served on the Virginia Law Review.

WALTER H. MEYER was Associate Director for Food Products Development with the Procter & Gamble Company from 1948 until his retirement in 1987. Since then, he has been a consultant to the food industry on food labeling and safety issues. He has served as chairman or member of a variety of food industry technical committees or advisory groups throughout his career. Mr. Meyer was a member of the National Academy of Sciences food industry liaison panel, the American Health Foundation food industry liaison panel, and the U.S. industry group serving the Codex Alimentarius Commission. He holds a B.S. in chemical engineering from Michigan State University.

PATRICIA McGRATH MORRIS is Director of Research at Public Voice for Food and Health Policy in Washington, D.C., where she has been on the staff since 1988. She recently published *Lean on Labels: A Survey of Meat and Poultry Products in Today's Marketplace* and *Blinded by "Lite": How*

Consumers View Food Labeling Claims. Ms. Morris was founder and co-owner of Forlenza-McGrath Associates, a radio news service firm for members of Congress and political candidates. Patty holds a B.A. from Trinity College and an M.S. in nutrition from Cornell University.

LAURA S. SIMS is Dean of the College of Human Ecology at the University of Maryland at College Park. Prior to this appointment, she was Administrator of the Human Nutrition Information Service at the U.S. Department of Agriculture (USDA). Before joining USDA, Laura was Professor of Nutrition in Public Health and Senior Research Associate in the Institute of Policy Research and Evaluation at Pennsylvania State University. Dr. Sims has served as Editor of the *Journal of Nutrition Education* and Chair of the Council on Research of the American Dietetic Association. Laura holds a B.S. in nutrition and family studies from Pennsylvania State University, an M.P.H. in nutrition from the University of Michigan, and a Ph.D. in Nutrition from Michigan State University.

BAILUS WALKER, Jr., is Dean of the College of Public Health at the Health Sciences Center of the University of Oklahoma, Oklahoma City. Before moving to Oklahoma, he was Professor of Public Health Policy at the State University of New York at Albany. Dr. Walker was the first non-physician to be appointed Commissioner of Public Health in Massachusetts, Chairman of the Massachusetts State Board of Health, and Michigan State Director of Public Health. Bailus is a member of the Institute of Medicine, has served on several IOM committees, and is a past president of the American Public Health Association. He holds a B.S. in biology and chemistry from Kentucky University, an M.P.H. in occupational and environmental health from the University of Michigan, and a Ph.D. in occupational and environmental health from the University of Minnesota.

NANCY S. WELLMAN is Professor in the Department of Dietetics and Nutrition, College of Health, Florida International University, in Miami. Prior to joining the faculty, she was the Nutrition Division Director and Adjunct Assistant Professor for the Department of Pediatrics at the University of Miami Mailman Center for Child Development. Dr. Wellman, a registered dietitian, is a past President of the 62,000-member American Dietetic Association. She holds a B.S. in home economics education from the State University College of New York at Buffalo, an M.S. in nutrition from Columbia University's Institute of Nutrition, and a Ph.D. in education from the University of Miami.

DONNA V. PORTER is Project Director of the Committee on State Food Labeling. She is a Specialist in Life Sciences at the Congressional Research Service (CRS) of the Library of Congress in Washington, D.C., where she has worked since 1980. Dr. Porter served as project director for the 1990 study by the Committee on the Nutrition Components of Food Labeling which issued *Nutrition Labeling: Issues and Directions for the 1990s*, for which she received the FDA Commissioner's Special Citation Award in 1991. Prior to joining the Library, Donna was a Fellow at the National Nutrition Consortium in Washington and a Congressional Science Fellow assigned to the Science Policy Research Division of CRS. She holds a B.S. in food and nutrition from the State University of New York at Plattsburgh, and a Ph.D. in human nutrition with a minor in political science from the Ohio State University.

ROBERT O. EARL is a Staff Officer with the Food and Nutrition Board (FNB) working with the Committee on State Food Labeling and on other FNB studies. He was previously Staff Officer for the study by the Committee on the Nutrition Components of Food Labeling, which issued *Nutrition Labeling: Issues and Directions for the 1990s*. Prior to joining the Institute of Medicine, Mr. Earl was Administrator of Government Affairs for the American Dietetic Association in Washington, D.C., covering food, nutrition, and health issues. Previously, Bob was statewide nutrition consultant for adult health, chronic disease, and health promotion programs with the Texas Department of Health. He holds a B.S. in human nutrition from the University of Michigan, an M.P.H. in public health nutrition from the University of North Carolina at Chapel Hill, and has begun working on a doctorate at the Institute for Public Policy at George Mason University, Fairfax, Virginia.

BARBARA L. MATOS is Project Assistant of the Committee on State Food Labeling. She was previously Project Assistant for Food and Nutrition Board studies by the Committee on Evaluation of the Safety of Fishery Products and the Committee on Evaluation of USDA Streamlined Inspection System for Cattle. Prior to joining the Institute of Medicine, Mrs. Matos was Educational Programs Coordinator at the American College of Radiology in Reston, Virginia, and Administrator of the Cancer Education Office of the University of Rochester Cancer Center. She holds a B.S. in sociology and an M.S. in health professions education from the University of Rochester.

Index

Adequacy of implementation of FDCA
  charge to Committee, 2, 30
  committee deliberations on, 73-80
  compliance and, 5
  consumer interest group views
    on, 72-73
  criteria for determining, 4-7, 31, 80-82
  definition of adequate, 4, 64, 69-70,
    73, 80
  enforcement and, 4, 5, 74, 77-78, 81,
    142-144
  evaluation process, 5-6, 30-33, 73-76
  industry views on, 71-72
  nonregulatory indicators of, 5, 76-78
  regulations and, 4, 5, 74, 81
  State and local views on, 69-71
  State requirements as indicators, 78-80
Administrative Conference of the United
    States, 66
Administrative Procedure Act, 66, 67
Adulteration of foods
  defined, 126, 128, 134
  economic, 87, 88, 125, 134
  honey, 119
  poi, 125
  pre-1900 concerns, 37
  1900–1940, 41
  noninjurious, 42
Advisory Committee on the Food and Drug
    Administration, 143-144
Advisory opinions
  catfish, 21, 123
  defined, 67

documents accorded status of, 76-77
  implementation of FDCA with, 6-7,
    66-67
  procedure for obtaining, 76
  significance given by Committee to, 6-7
  wild rice, 126
Alabama requirements
  discrepancies between Federal require-
    ments and, 196
  honey, 119 n.10
  materials provided to Committee, 184
  misleading containers, 93
  prominence of required information,
    100
Alaska requirements
  artificial colors, flavors, and
    preservatives, 130 n.12
  common or usual name, 121
  discrepancies between Federal require-
    ments and, 196
  materials provided to Committee, 184
  misleading containers, 93
Animal Drugs Amendments of 1968, 47
Apples, 196-201
Aquaculture products, 10, 121
Arizona Consumers Council, 113, 196
Arizona requirements
  artificial colors, flavors, and preserva-
    tives, 130 n.12, 131
  bottled water, 116 n.8
  common or usual names, 110
  discrepancies between Federal require-
    ments and, 196

Arizona requirements, *continued*
  materials provided to Committee, 185
  placement of required information,
    101 n.6
Arkansas requirements
  artificial colors, flavors, and preserva-
    tives, 130 n.12
  common or usual names, 121
  discrepancies between Federal require-
    ments and, 196
  honey, 119 n.10
  materials provided to Committee, 184
  placement of required information,
    99 n.1, 100 n.3
Armour meat products, 40
Artificial flavorings, colorings, or chemical
    preservatives, 29, 44
  in bulk foods, 131
  common or usual names, 127, 128,
    131, 134-135
  in dairy products, 130
  discrepancies between Federal and
    State requirements, 129, 197, 200
  enforcement activity, 128, 132-133
  exemptions from declaration, 134-135
  Federal requirements, 127-132
  food innovations and, 59
  industry opposition to legislation, 41
  mixtures of preservatives, 131
  prohibitions in specific foods, 130
  prominence of required information,
    101
  quantity restrictions, 131
  in restaurant/bakery foods, 132, 133
  safety regulation, 47
  in specific foods, 130
  State requirements, 129-133, 134
  sulfites, 128, 129, 132, 133, 196,
    200, 201
Aseptic processing, 45, 48
Association of Food and Drug Officials
    (AFDO), 31, 32
  membership, 55-56
  Model Bottled Water Regulation, 18,
    116-117, 217
  purpose, 39-40
  Uniform State Food, Drug, and
    Cosmetic Bill, 8, 55, 58
  views on factors influencing adequacy
    of implementation, 69, 143

Association of Official Agricultural
    Chemists, 39
Association of Official Analytical
    Chemists, 39
Association of State and Territorial Health
    Officials, 32

Beverages
  colors, flavors, and preservatives, 131,
    197, 199, 200
  fruit, 112
  nonalcoholic, 101
  powdered mixes, 93
  water component in flavored
    products, 116
Blended foods, 44, 100-101, 123
Borden Foods, 153
Bottled water labeling
  AFDO Model Regulation, 18,
    116-117, 216
  carbonation, 117
  case study, 209-217
  Committee conclusions, 9, 18, 117, 217
  common or usual name, 18, 110, 111-
    112, 115, 116, 209-210
  Congressional scrutiny, 213-217
  discrepancies between Federal and
    State requirements, 196-200
  distilled water, 212
  false and misleading claims, 18, 117
  Federal requirements, 204, 209
  Good Manufacturing Practice for, 116,
    212-213
  identifying terms, 115
  industry perspective on, 106
  mineral water, 116, 209
  recalls, 209, 214
  spring water, 89, 112, 212
  standards of identity, 18
  standards of quality, 104, 111, 115, 116,
    209, 210-213
  State requirements, 70, 89, 110, 111-
    112, 116, 204, 217
  water component in flavored beverage
    products, 116
  well water, 111, 212
Bulk foods, 43, 127, 196, 197, 199
Burditt, George, 145
Bureau of Enforcement Guideline, 128

California requirements
  artificial colors and flavors, 130, 131
  bottled water, 70, 110, 116 n.8
  common or usual names, 110
  container fill, 13, 92, 94, 95, 97
  discrepancies between Federal
    requirements and, 196
  honey, 119 n.10
  materials provided to Committee, 185
  olive and vegetable oils, 123
  placement of required information,
    99 n.1, 100
Candy, 88, 92
Caramel, 128
Case law
  *Hobby Industry Association of America,
    Inc. v. Younger,* 94
  U.S. v. 30 Cases, 105
  U.S. v. 46 Cases, 98
  U.S. v. 62 Cases, 105
  U.S. v. 70 Gross Bottles, 99
  U.S. v. 88 Cases, 88
  U.S. v. 95 Barrels, 88
  U.S. v. 116 Boxes, 92
  U.S. v. 174 Cases (Delson Thin
    Mints), 92
  U.S. v. 274 Boxes, 99
  U.S. v. Antonio Corrao Corp., 129
  U.S. v. Caraldo, 92
  U.S. v. Sullivan, 129
Catsup, 130
Center for Science in the Public Interest
  (CSPI), views on adequacy of
  FDCA implementation, 72, 96, 102,
  133, 149
Cereals, 93
Cholesterol labeling terminology, 53
Cider, cider vinegar, and other vinegar
  products, 9, 18, 88, 100, 110, 112, 117-
  118, 130, 197, 198, 199, 208
Citrus products, 10, 18-19, 44, 111, 118-119,
  131, 196
Code of Federal Regulations (CFR), Title
  21, Parts and Sections (§)
  Part 1, 67
  §1.20, 58
  §1.21, 58
  §1.24, 88
  §10.85, 5, 67, 68, 76
  §10.90, 68, 77
  §70.3(f), 127

Part 74, 128
§101.1, 58, 98
§101.2, 58, 98
§101.3, 58, 98, 107, 112
§101.4, 58
§101.5, 58
§101.10, 129
§101.15, 58
§101.18, 58, 88, 95
§101.22, 58, 127-128, 131, 133, 135, 136
§101.35, 135
§101.100, 127, 128
§101.105, 58, 95
Part 102, 17, 58, 59, 66, 89, 107, 108,
  112, 113-114, 120, 204
§103.14, 58, 104
§103.35, 106, 204
§105.62, 135
§105.65, 135
Part 129, 116, 204, 212-213, 217
Part 139, 124
Part 161, 206
§168.40, 206
§172.510, 127
§172.515, 127
§182.10, 127
§182.60, 127
§182.3739 – .3862, 128
Part 184, 127
preambles to regulations, 6, 7, 66,
  67, 76
Coffee and tea, 44, 48, 93
Color Additive Amendments, 47, 126
Colorado requirements
  artificial colors, flavors, and
    preservatives, 131
  honey, 119 n.10
  discrepancies between Federal require-
    ments and, 196
  materials provided to Committee, 185
  placement of required information,
    99 n.1
Common or usual names, 29, 59
  blended oils, 123-124
  CFR list, 108
  delay in establishment of, 90
  Federal requirements, 107-110
  flavorings, 127
  imitation, alternative, and substitute
    food products, 109-110
  implementing regulations, 89, 107-108

Common or usual names, *continued*
  overlap with standards of quality
    and identity, 7, 80, 89, 110
  petition process, 17, 90, 107, 108-109
  preservatives, 128
  purpose of, 88-89
  rulemaking on, 66
  for specific foods, 17-22, 89, 114-122
  State requirements, 110-112
  violations, 77
  see also individual foods; FDCA Section
    403(i)(1)
Compliance Policy Guides, 7, 20, 76, 121,
    122, 124
Connecticut requirements
  artificial colors, flavors, and
    preservatives, 130 n.12, 132, 133
  bottled water, 110, 116 n.8
  cider products, 118 n.9
  common or usual names, 110
  discrepancies between Federal
    requirements and, 196
  honey, 119 n.10
  materials provided to Committee, 185
  misleading containers, 94
  preservatives, 129
  prominence of required information, 99
    n.1, 100 nn.2, 4, 101
Constitutional Convention of 1789, 37-38
Consumer education, 28, 51, 54
Consumer interest groups
  views on adequacy of FDA implementa-
    tion of FDCA, 71-72, 89, 96, 102, 113,
    133-134
  see also individual groups
Consumer Product Safety Commission, 150
Container fill, *see* Misleading containers;
    Slack fill; Standards of quality
    and fill
Crawford, Bob, 142-143
Crepe labeling, 104, 106

Dairy products, *see* Milk, milk products,
    and other dairy products
Delaware requirements
  bottled water, 116 n.8
  discrepancies between Federal
    requirements and, 196
  prominence of required information,
    99 n.1

Dietary recommendations, and
    food descriptors, 109
Dietary supplements, 52
Dingell, John D., 213-214
District of Columbia, food and drug
    legislation, 37

Economic costs of nonuniformity, 23, 25
  to consumers, 153
  information requested on, 33
  interstate commerce and, 43, 44, 47, 50
  legal confrontations, 153, 156
  monitoring of State legislative and
    regulatory activities, 153, 154-155
  practical value of uniform labeling,
    157-159
  product negotiations with individual
    States, 153, 155-156
  product retrieval, relabeling, and
    scrapping, 154, 156-157
Eggs, 88, 92
Enforcement of Federal requirements
  and adequacy of FDCA implemen-
    tation, 4, 5, 74, 77-78, 81
  concerns about, 23-24, 90, 142-144
  court actions, 65; *see also* Case law
  defined, 74
  evaluation of, 5, 77-78
  FDA priorities, 74
  fiscal and resource constraints on,
    23-24, 74, 78, 142, 144, 145, 148,
    159, 215-216
  formal remedies, 146
  informal remedies, 44, 74-75, 146-147
  under multiple sections of FDCA, 77,
    86, 87
  NLEA mandate, 28, 54
  prior notification requirement, 29,
    145, 146
  process, 24, 144-147
  sanctions, 44
  State concerns about, 32
  uniform code for, 148
Enzyme technology, 45
Europe, standardization of labeling, 158-159
Executive Order 12612, 68, 152
Extrusion of carbohydrate and protein
    foods, 45

Fair Packaging and Labeling Act of 1966
  implementing regulations, 47
  nonfunctional slack fill provision, 12,
    14, 92, 97
  preemption of State regulation, 47
  statement of identity, 107
Federal Food, Drug, and Cosmetic Act
  of 1938 (FDCA)
  advisory opinions and implementation
    of, 66-67
  amendments, 47, 52, 65, 116, 126
  automatic adoption by States, 55, 70-71
  court enforcement actions, 65
  enactment, 3, 27
  enforcement by States, 29
  food defined, 43-44
  interstate commerce jurisdiction, 47
  overlap in provisions of, 1, 86
  provisions studied, 1-2, 28
  purpose of misbranding provisions,
    3, 46
  rulemaking authority and activities,
    65, 66
  violations of labeling provisions, 46
  see also Adequacy of implementation
    of FDCA
FD&C Yellow Dye No. 5, 128
FDCA Section 201(f), 43-44
FDCA Section 401, 12, 15, 16, 19, 20, 91,
  92, 103, 120, 210, 211
FDCA Section 402, 87, 88, 128, 136
FDCA Section 403(a)(1), 4, 77, 80
FDCA Section 403(b), 1, 11-12, 28, 87-90
  adequacy of implementation, 9, 77
  case law, 88
  Committee conclusions and recommen-
    dations, 9, 12, 90
  consumer perspective on, 11-12, 89
  enforcement of, 89
  exempted foods, 88
  Federal and State requirements
    compared, 11-12, 87-89
  industry perspective on, 11-12, 89
  intent of, 11, 87-88
  nomenclature issues, 59, 90
  overlap with FDCA Section 403(i)(1),
    11-12, 87
  preemption date, 29, 63
  see also Food sold under the name of
    another food; Section
    403(i)(1)

FDCA Section 403(c)
  preemption date, 29, 63
FDCA Section 403(d), 28
  Committee conclusions and recommen-
    dations, 9, 13-14, 96-97
  consumer perspective on, 13, 96
  enforcement of, 95, 97
  Federal and State requirements
    compared, 12-14, 72-73, 90-92
  implementation of, 9, 91-92
  industry perspective on, 13, 95
  packaging innovations and potential
    violations, 59
  preemption date, 29, 63
  related statutory sections, 92
  see also Misleading container; Slack
    fill
FDCA Section 403(e), 4, 29, 77, 80
FDCA Section 403(f), 1, 14-15, 28, 97-103
  case law, 98-99
  Committee conclusions and recommen-
    dations, 9, 14-15, 102-103
  consumer perspective on, 14, 102
  Federal and State requirements
    compared, 14-15, 97-101
  implementing regulations, 14, 98
  industry perspective on, 14, 102
  packaging innovations and potential
    violations, 59
  preemption date, 29, 63
  see also Prominence of required
    information
FDCA Section 403(g), 29, 87
FDCA Section 403(h), 1, 15-16, 28,
  103-106
  case law, 104-105
  Committee conclusions and recommen-
    dations, 9, 16, 106
  consumer perspective on, 106
  Federal and State requirements
    compared, 15-16, 72-73, 103-105
  industry perspective on, 105-106
  preemption date, 29, 63
  related statutory provisions, 15, 92, 101
  see also Standards of quality and fill
FDCA Section 403(i)(1), 2, 16-21, 28, 107-
  126, 209-210
  adequacy of implementation, 9-11, 77
  Committee conclusions and recommen-
    dations, 9-11, 17, 113-126
  consumer perspective on, 17, 113

FDCA Section 403(i)(1), *continued*
  distinction from FDCA Section 403(b), 87
  enforcement of, 17
  Federal and State requirements compared, 16-17, 107-112
  industry perspective on, 17, 112-113
  nomenclature issues, 59
  overlap with other statutory provisions, 11-12, 110
  petition process, 17, 108-109
  preemption date, 29, 63, 80
  see also Common or usual name
FDCA Section 403(i)(2), 4, 28, 77, 80
FDCA Section 403(k), 2, 22-23, 28, 59, 126-136
  case law, 129
  Committee conclusions and recommendations, 11, 22-23, 134-136
  consumer perspective on, 22, 133-134
  exemptions from, 127
  Federal and State requirements compared, 16-17, 22-23, 126-133
  implementing regulations, 127-128
  industry perspective on, 22, 133
  preemption date, 29, 63
  related statutory provisions, 16, 101
  see also Artificial flavorings, colorings, or chemical preservatives
FDCA Section 403(q), 29
FDCA Section 403(r), 29
FDCA Section 410, 116
FDCA Section 701(a), 65
FDCA Section 706(a), 65
Federal Register notices, use of, 76
Federal Trade Commission, 3, 52
Fish List, The 10, 21, 67, 120, 122
Fish
  catfish, 10, 121, 123, 198
  common or usual names, 120-121
  discrepancies between Federal and State requirements, 196, 204
  halibut, 121, 199, 201, 204
  misleading containers, 93
  nonstandardized products, 59, 89
  red snapper, 121
  substitutes, 10, 121-122
Florida requirements
  artificial colors, flavors, and preservatives, 130 n.12
  bottled water, 111, 116 n.8

citrus code, 18-19, 69, 111
common or usual names, 19, 111, 116 n.8
discrepancies between Federal requirements and, 196
enforcement concerns, 142-143
honey, 119 n.10
materials provided to Committee, 185
misleading containers, 93
prominence of required information, 100 n.3
standards of fill of container, 105
Foam-mat drying, 44-45
Food, statutory definition, 43
Food additives
  guidance on safety studies, 67
  legislation, 126-127
  see also Artificial flavorings, colorings, or chemical preservatives
Food Additives Amendment of 1958, 47, 126
Food and Drug Administration, 3
  authority under NLEA, 54
  cooperative relationship with States, 23, 24, 142, 147-149
  expenditures on food activities, 56, 57
  Fish List, The 67
  food program categories, 56
  joint initiatives with States, 56-57
  National, Regional, and State Telecommunications Network (NRSTEN), 31, 32
  preemption policy, 68-69, 151-153
  Red Book, The 67
  regulatory authority, 27, 28
  review and reform of food labeling, 52, 53
Food descriptors, 28, 52, 54, 102, 106, 109
Food industry
  concerns about nonuniformity of regulations, 27-28
  protectionist requirements, 69
  support of legislation by, 42, 54
  views on adequacy of FDA implementation of FDCA, 71-72, 89, 95, 102, 105-106, 112-113, 133
Food labeling
  Federal and State requirements compared, 7-23, 85-136
  value of uniformity in, 39

Food labels
    criticisms of, 4, 52
Food labels
    format, 14, 52, 53, 54, 102, 104
    prior approval, 43
Food production and marketing
    before 1900, 36
    1900–1940, 40
    1940–1970, 44-46
    1970–1990, 48-50
    diverting network, 49-50
    innovations in, 44-45
Food products, evolution of, 3, 36, 40, 49
Food safety
    common or usual names and, 21, 113,
        122, 128, 135-136
    guidance on studies, 67
    regulation of, 41, 44, 47
    warning statements on labels, 22, 134,
        136
Food sold under the name of another food,
    29, 77, 87-90
    see also FDCA Section 403(b)
Fortification/enrichment of foods, 46, 52
Freshly prepared and catered products, 49
Fruit juices, 19, 110, 111, 118, 200
Frozen desserts, 100, 112, 199, 200, 201
Frozen foods, 40, 44, 199

Gelatin desserts, 40, 91-92
Georgia requirements
    artificial colors, flavors, and preserva-
        tives, 130 n.12
    common or usual names, 111, 125
    discrepancies between Federal
        requirements and, 196
    honey, 119 n.10
    materials provided to Committee, 185
    misleading containers, 95
    Vidalia onions, 10, 21, 125, 196
Good Manufacturing Practice, 116, 212-213
Grading systems, 19, 118, 119, 123,
    196, 197
Grain mixtures, 198
Great Atlantic and Pacific Tea Company
    (A&P), 36, 40
Grits, 198
Grocery Manufacturers of America (GMA),
    views on FDCA implementation,
    72, 89, 105, 106-107, 113, 145, 153

Grocery stores
    chains, 36, 40
    self-serve, 40

Harden, Betty, 143
Hawaii requirements
    bottled water, 112, 116 n.8
    common or usual names, 112
    discrepancies between Federal require-
        ments and, 197
    materials provided to Committee, 185
    oriental noodle products, 124
    poi, 20, 125, 152, 197
    standards of identity, 124, 125
Health and organic foods, 45
Health and nutrition claims, 4, 28, 29
    petition mechanism under NLEA, 54
    regulation of, 51, 52-54
Health Research and Health Services Act,
    Proxmire Amendment, 52
Honey, 10, 19, 100, 119-120, 196-201,
    205-206
House Committee on Energy and
    Commerce's Subcommittee on
    Oversight and Investigations, 116,
    209, 213
Hutt, Peter Barton, 64
Hypoallergenic foods, 135

Idaho requirements
    discrepancies between Federal require-
        ments and, 197
    materials provided to Committee, 186
    prominence of required information,
        99 n.1, 100 nn.2, 3
Identity labeling of food, 98
Illinois requirements
    discrepancies between Federal require-
        ments and, 197
    materials provided to Committee, 186
Imitation foods, 29, 52, 63
    defined, 109
    Federal labeling requirements, 109-110,
        121-122, 197
    flavors, 199
    seafood, 121-122
Implementation of FDCA
    advisory opinions as means of, 6-7,
        66-67, 74

Implementation of FDCA, *continued*
  court enforcement actions, 65
  historical approach of FDA, 65-69
  informal communications and, 6, 67-68
  preemption policy of FDA, 68-69
  rulemaking used for, 66
  see also Adequacy of implementation of
    FDCA; Code of Federal
    Regulations
Indiana requirements
  discrepancies between Federal require-
    ments and, 197
  materials provided to Committee, 186
  placement of required information,
    99-100
Industry, *see* Food industry
Infant foods, 135
Infant Formula Act, 52
Information panel, 98
Ingredient statement, 28, 29, 52
  artificial colors, flavors, and preserva-
    tives in, 134, 135
  blended oils, 123-124
  importance to consumers, 59
  reforms, 53, 54
  trade secrets and, 134
  violations, 77
International Bottled Water Association
  (IBWA), 213
Interstate commerce, 43, 44, 47, 49-50,
  58-59, 146, 150, 154
Intrastate commerce, 145, 146
Iowa requirements
  cider products, 118 n.9
  discrepancies between Federal require-
    ments and, 197
  honey, 119 n.10
  materials provided to Committee, 186
  prominence of required information,
    99 n.1, 100 n.5, 101 n.7
Irradiation of foods, 48, 201

Kansas requirements
  artificial colors, flavors, and
    preservatives, 130 n.12
  discrepancies between Federal require-
    ments and, 197
  honey, 119 n.10
  materials provided to Committee, 186
  prominence of required information,
    99 n.1

Kellogg Company, 153
Kentucky requirements
  artificial colors, flavors, and
    preservatives, 130 n.12
  discrepancies between Federal require-
    ments and, 197
  materials provided to Committee, 187
Kessler, David, 110, 143
Kraft General Foods, Inc., 71, 113

Land O'Lakes, 153
Legislation, *see specific statutes*
Life expectancy, 41
Louisiana requirements
  artificial colors, flavors, and
    preservatives, 130 n.12
  bottled water, 116 n.8
  discrepancies between Federal require-
    ments and, 197
  honey, 119 n.10
  materials provided to Committee, 187

Macaroni, 130, 199
Madison, James, 38
Maine requirements
  artificial colors, flavors, and
    preservatives, 130, 132
  bottled water, 116 n.8
  cider products, 112, 118
  common or usual names, 112, 118, 122
  discrepancies between Federal require-
    ments and, 197
  materials provided to Committee, 187
  seafood, 122
Manufacturer's name and address, 29, 77
Maple products, 10, 19, 100-101, 112, 123,
  197, 198, 199, 201, 206
Maryland requirements
  artificial colors, flavors, and
    preservatives, 132
  bottled water, 116 n.8
  common or usual names, 122
  discrepancies between Federal require-
    ments and, 197
  enforcement concerns, 142-143
  materials provided to Committee, 187
  seafood, 122, 132
  standards of fill of container, 105

Massachusetts requirements
  artificial colors, flavors, and
    preservatives, 130 n.12
  cider products, 118 n.9
  common or usual names, 121
  discrepancies between Federal require-
    ments and, 197
  materials provided to Committee, 188
  prominence of required information,
    99 n.1, 100, 101 n.7
Meat and poultry products
  common or usual name, 110
  inspection programs, 54-55
  nutrition labeling, 51-52
  regulation of, 43, 47-48
Meat Inspection Act of 1907, 43
Membrane processing systems, 45
Michigan requirements
  artificial colors, flavors, and
    preservatives, 130 n.12, 133
  cider products, 112, 118
  common or usual names, 112, 118
  discrepancies between Federal require-
    ments and, 197
  materials provided to Committee, 188
  misleading containers, 93
  prominence of required information,
    99 n.1
Microbiological standards, 19, 119
Microwave cooking, 48
Milk, milk products, and other dairy
    products
  artificial colors, flavors, and
    preservatives, 129, 130, 135
  Committee conclusions, 10, 19-20, 120
  discrepancies between Federal and
    State requirements, 19-20, 129,
    196-201
  instant and dried milk powders, 44, 45
  monitoring of legislative activities, 154
  packaging innovations, 36
  pasteurization, 36
  product negotiations, 155
  prominence of label information,
    14, 99-100
  standards of identity, 20, 112, 120
  substitutes, 14, 99-100, 154, 201
Minnesota requirements
  artificial colors, flavors, and
    preservatives, 130 n.12, 131, 133

  discrepancies between Federal require-
    ments and, 197
  honey, 119 n.10
  materials provided to Committee, 188
  misleading containers, 94
  prominence of required information,
    99 n.1, 100, 101
  standards of quality and fill, 101, 105
  wild rice, 125
Misleading containers, 29, 37, 59
  downsizing or package shorting, 70, 93,
    96, 198
  case law on, 91-92, 96
  deceptive packaging, 90, 198
  evaluation criteria, 92
  Federal requirements, 90-92
  slack fill, nonfunctional, 47, 90, 92, 94,
    95, 196
  State regulation of, 12-14, 70, 72-73, 91,
    93-95, 96, 97
  see also FDCA Section 403(d)
Mississippi requirements
  bottled water, 116 n.8
  common or usual names, 121
  discrepancies between Federal require-
    ments and, 198
  honey, 119 n.10
  materials provided to Committee, 188
  prominence of required information,
    99 n.1, 100
Missouri requirements
  discrepancies between Federal require-
    ments and, 198
  materials provided to Committee, 188
  prominence of required information,
    100 n.2
Monosodium glutamate, 127, 132, 133-134,
    135-136, 197
Montana requirements
  bottled water, 116 n.8
  discrepancies between Federal require-
    ments and, 198
  materials provided to Committee, 188
  prominence of required information,
    100 n.4

National Association of Attorneys
    General, 32
National Association of Consumer Affairs
    Administrators, 31

National Association of State Departments
   of Agriculture, 31
National Association of State Directors of
   Agriculture, 32
National Conference of Weights
   and Measures, 31
National Food Processors Association
   (NFPA), 150, 153
National Frozen Pizza Institute (NFPI),
   95, 102
National Primary Drinking Water
   Standards, 116
National, Regional, and State Telecom-
   unications Network (NRSTEN),
   31,32
Nebraska requirements
   discrepancies between Federal require-
      ments and, 198
   materials provided to Committee, 188
Net weight statement, 29, 47, 91, 94, 95
Nevada requirements
   common or usual names, 112
   discrepancies between Federal require-
      ments and, 198
   honey, 119 n.10
   materials provided to Committee, 188
   prominence of required information,
      99 n.1
New Hampshire requirements
   artificial colors, flavors, and
      preservatives, 130 n.12
   cider products, 118 n.9
   discrepancies between Federal require-
      ments and, 198
   honey, 119 n.10
   materials provided to Committee, 188
   prominence of required information,
      100 n.2, 3, 101 n.7
New Jersey requirements
   bottled water, 116 n.8
   discrepancies between Federal require-
      ments and, 198
   honey, 119 n.10
   materials provided to Committee, 188
   misleading containers, 94
   prominence of required information,
      101 n.7
New Mexico requirements
   artificial colors, flavors, and
      preservatives, 130 n.12

discrepancies between Federal requirements and, 198
honey, 119 n.10
materials provided to Committee, 189
pine nuts, 20, 124
New York requirements
   bottled water, 70
   cider products, 118 n.9
   discrepancies between Federal require-
      ments and, 199
   honey, 119 n.10
   maple syrup, 123
   materials provided to Committee, 189
   misleading containers, 72-73, 93
   olive and vegetable oils, 123-124
   prominence of required information,
      99 n.1, 100, 101 n.7
   standards of fill of container, 105
Niles, Ray, 89, 111
Nonorganic solvent techniques, 48
North Carolina requirements
   discrepancies between Federal require-
      ments and, 199
   materials provided to Committee, 189
North Dakota requirements
   artificial colors, flavors, and
      preservatives, 130 n.12
   bottled water, 116 n.8
   discrepancies between Federal require-
      ments and, 199
   materials provided to Committee, 189
   prominence of required information,
      100 n.3
Nutrient claims, *see* Health and
   nutrition claims
Nutrient content information, 28, 29, 53, 54
   rulemaking on, 66
Nutrition
   deficiency diseases, 41
   and health, 46, 50-51
Nutrition labeling
   amendment of FDCA and provisions
      for, 52
   appropriateness review of, 3-4, 52
   dietary recommendations and, 51
   mandatory, 28, 51, 53, 54
   reform efforts, 52-54
   preemption schedule, 29
   prevalence and adequacy of, 51-52
   voluntary, 28, 51, 54

Nutrition Labeling and Education Act
of 1990 (NLEA)
ambiguities in, 16, 106
enactment, 1, 28, 54
enforcement authority under, 29, 40, 74,
141, 144-147
exemption policies, 68, 142
FDA authority under, 28
overlap with FDCA, 1
purpose of, 63, 141
reforms addressed by, 4
requirements of, 28, 54
Section 4, 144-146
Section 6, 28, 63, 64-65, 74, 85, 136
Section 7, 136
Section 403A(b), 150, 151
study mandate to IOM, 29-30, 64,
85, 165-166
see also Preemption of State and
local regulations
Nuts, 11, 20, 124, 196, 198, 199, 207

Ohio requirements
artificial colors, flavors, and
preservatives, 130 n.12, 131
bottled water, 116 n.8
cider products, 118 n.9
discrepancies between Federal requirements and, 199
honey, 119 n.10
materials provided to Committee,
189-190
Oklahoma requirements
artificial colors, flavors, and
preservatives, 130 n.12
bottled water, 116 n.8
discrepancies between Federal requirements and, 199
honey, 119 n.10
materials provided to Committee, 191
Oleomargarine/margarine, 99-100, 131,
199, 200
Olive and vegetable oils, 44
adulteration, 129, 130
Committee findings and conclusions
on, 10, 20, 123-124
discrepancies between Federal and
State requirements, 123-124, 196,
199, 200, 207
prominence regulations, 100

Onion rings, 59
Onions, 21, 199, *see also* Vidalia onions
Open dating, 52
Oranges, 131
Orange juice, 69, 88, 89
Oregon requirements
common or usual names, 121
discrepancies between Federal require-
ments and, 199
materials provided to Committee, 191
prominence of required information,
100 n.3
Oriental noodles, 10, 20, 112, 124, 197
Oysters, canned, 75, 105, 196, 197

Packaging
branded, 40
innovations, 36, 44, 45-46, 59
and marketability, 3
materials, 40, 45
microbiological growth control, 49
misleading containers, 59, 90-91
plastics, 45-46, 48-49
retort pouch, 45
Uneeda Biscuit, 36
see also Misleading containers
Peanut spreads, 89
Pecans, 196, 198, 207
Pellagra, 41
Pennsylvania requirements
artificial colors, flavors, and
preservatives, 130, 131
cider products, 118 n.9, 130
discrepancies between Federal requirements and, 200
materials provided to Committee, 191
prominence of required information,
99 n.1, 100, 101
Pepsico – Frito Lay, 153
Pesticides Amendment of 1954, 47
Petition process, 23, 25, 68-69, 142,
144-147, 149-153
Piggly-Wiggly, 40
Pine nuts, 11, 20, 124, 198
Poi, 11, 20, 112, 125, 152, 197
Potato chips, 59, 89
Poultry inspection program, 43, 47
Poultry Product Inspection Act of 1957, 47
Preemption of State and local regulations
conditions for, 29, 63
exemption policy, 24, 68, 150

Preemption of State and local regulations,
    continued
    under Fair Packaging and Labeling Act
        of 1966, 47
    FDA policy, 68-69, 151-153
    impact evaluation, 31
    implementation problems, 38
    industry support of, 42, 54
    on meat and poultry inspections, 47-48
    origin of doctrine of, 37-38
    petition process for exemptions, 23-25,
        32, 142, 144, 149-153
    schedule for, 1, 28, 54, 63-64
    strictness of requirements as a
        consideration, 4, 75, 81, 133
    uniformity without, 39-40
Principal display panel, 98
    flavors on, 127
    identity labeling, 98
Prior label approval, 47
Processed foods, 47
Processed Products Inspection
    Improvement Act of 1986, 47
Procter & Gamble Company, 153
Produce, nutrition labeling of, 28, 54,
    196-199, 201
Prominence of required information, 29, 47,
    54, 59
    blended products, 100-101
    colors, flavors, and preservatives, 101
    dairy product substitutes, 99-100
    Federal requirements, 98-99
    State requirements, 99-101
    see also FDCA Section 403(f)
Public health
    before 1900, 37
    1900-1940, 41-42
    1940-1970, 46
    1970-1990, 50-51
Public Voice for Food and Health
    Policy, 149
Puerto Rico requirements
    materials provided to Committee, 191
Pure Food and Drugs Act of 1906, 3, 27,
    41, 42-43, 86, 87, 88, 126

Quaker Oats Company, 95, 153

Recycling, 45
Red Book, The, 67
Reference values, 53

Refrigerated prepared foods, 48
Regulation of misbranded food
    before 1900, 37-40
    1900-1940, 42-44
    1940-1970, 47-48
    1970-1990, 51-54
    current Federal and State roles, 54-58
    exemptions to protect local interests, 58
    historical context for, 3-4, 35-54
    increasing use of rulemaking, 66
    interstate commerce and, 43, 44, 47, 50,
        58-59
    see also Code of Federal Regulations;
        Preemption of State and local regu-
        lations
Regulatory Amendments of 1948, 47
Restaurant/bakery foods, 132, 133
Rhode Island requirements
    artificial colors, flavors, and
        preservatives, 130, 132
    cider products, 118 n.9, 130
    discrepancies between Federal require-
        ments and, 200
    materials provided to Committee, 192
    olive and vegetable oils, 123
Rice, 200; *see also* Wild rice
RJR Nabisco, 153
Roosevelt, Theodore, 147-148

Safe Drinking Water Act, 116, 212
Safe Medical Devices Act of 1990, 65
Salad bars, 132, 133
Salt/sodium, 127
Sanitation, 37, 39, 41
Schreiber Foods, Inc., 95
Schultz, William, 64
Seafood, 20-21, 120-123
    artificial colors, flavors, and
        preservatives, 132, 200
    Committee findings and conclusions,
        10, 20-21, 120-123
    common or usual names, 20-21, 110,
        113, 120-122
    Federal requirements, 197
    finfish and shellfish, 113, 120-121
    misleading container, 93
    nutrition labeling, 28, 54
    State requirements, 93, 197
    surimi-based imitations and substitutes,
        10, 21, 121-122, 207
    see also Fish

Serving size, 53
Shank, Fred, 215-216
Silverglade, Bruce, 149
Slack fill, nonfunctional, 47, 90, 92, 94, 95
Sodium content and descriptors, 52
Soup mixes, 93
South Carolina requirements
  discrepancies between Federal require-
    ments and, 200
  materials provided to Committee, 192
South Dakota requirements
  artificial colors, flavors, and
    preservatives, 131
  common or usual names, 112
  discrepancies between Federal require-
    ments and, 200
  materials provided to Committee, 192
  prominence of required information,
    100 n.5, 101 n.6
Soybean cheese, 89, 111
Spaghetti sauce, 93
Specialty stores, 36, 49
Spices, 127, 134-135, 197, 198
Squalene, 129
Squibb, E.R., 39
Standards of identity, 3, 52, 104
  citrus products, 118-119
  defined, 107
  maple syrup, 123
  overlap with common or usual names,
    7, 80, 89, 110
  preemption date, 28, 29, 80
  reforms, 53, 66
  relationship to standards of quality,
    105-106, 110
Standards of quality and fill, 29, 54
  canned oysters, 75
  Federal requirements, 103-105, 197
  relationship to standards of identity,
    105-106, 110
  overlap with common or usual
    names, 110
  State requirements, 16, 94, 105, 197
  see also FDCA Section 403(d); Decep-
    tive packaging; Misleading contain-
    ers; Slack fill
Statements of Policy and Interpretation, 67
States
  authority under Pure Food and
    Drugs Act, 43

  automatic adoption of Federal statutes
    and regulations, 8, 55, 70-71
  categorization of requirements, 6
  cooperative relationship between
    FDA and, 23, 24, 142, 147-149
  concerns of, 80
  enforcement authority, 28, 29, 31,
    38-39, 40, 54, 141, 144-147
  funding for enforcement programs,
    48, 55
  joint initiatives with FDA, 56-57
  laws and regulations, 32, 37
  meat and poultry inspection
    programs, 54-55
  monitoring of legislative and regulatory
    activities, 154-155
  obsolete provisions, 58
  overlap with Federal activities, 7, 58, 72
  product negotiations between
    industry and, 155-156
  reasons for regulation by, 7, 8,
    55-56, 78-79
  regulations as indicators of FDCA
    implementation, 78-80, 81
  respondents to request for information,
    31, 173, 175-181
  review of requirements of,
    5, 79-80, 81
  role in regulation, 70, 72-73
  sovereignty, 37-38
  views on adequacy of FDA
    implementation of FDCA, 69-71
  see also individual states
Strawberries, 197
Substitute foods, 44, 52, 59
  Federal requirements, 109-110, 121-122
  prominence of label information,
    99-100
  seafood, 121-122
Sulfites, 128, 129, 132, 133, 196, 200, 201
Supercritical carbon dioxide, 48
Supermarkets, 36, 44, 49, 158
Surimi products, 10, 21, 112, 121-122,
  123, 197, 207

Tennessee requirements
  artificial colors, flavors, and
    preservatives, 132

Tennessee requirements, *continued*
    discrepancies between Federal require-
        ments and, 200
    materials provided to Committee, 192
Texas requirements
    artificial colors, flavors, and
        preservatives, 131, 132
    bottled water, 116 n.8
    discrepancies between Federal require-
        ments and, 200
    materials provided to Committee,
        192-193
    prominence of required information,
        100 n.4, 101 n.7
    seafood, 122
Texturized vegetable protein, 45, 59, 135
Thompson, Merrill, 71-72, 146
Tomato sauce, 130
Trade correspondence, 7, 67, 76, 91, 128
Tuna fish, canned, 93

U.S. Department of Agriculture, 3, 44, 53
    authority to preempt State
        regulation, 48
    Bureau of Chemistry, 39, 43
    Food Safety and Quality Service, 52
    grade standards, 119
    meat and poultry inspection budget, 55
U.S. Department of Health and
        Human Services, 53
Utah requirements
    common or usual names, 112
    discrepancies between Federal require-
        ments and, 200
    materials provided to Committee, 193
    prominence of required information,
        100 n.2

Vanilla, 130
Vanillin, 128, 130
Vegetable oils, *see* Olive and vegetable oils
Vending machines, 44
Vermont requirements
    artificial colors, flavors, and
        preservatives, 130 n.12
    common or usual names, 112
    discrepancies between Federal require-
        ments and, 201
    maple syrup, 123

materials provided to Committee, 193
    prominence of required information,
        99 n.1, 100 nn.3, 5,
Vidalia onions, 11, 21, 125, 196
Vinegar, *see* Cider, cider vinegar, and other
        vinegar products
Virginia requirements
    discrepancies between Federal require-
        ments and, 201
    materials provided to Committee, 193

Warning Letters, 75, 146
Warning statements on labels, 22, 134, 136
Washington requirements
    artificial colors, 130
    common or usual names, 121
    discrepancies between Federal require-
        ments and, 201
    honey, 119 n.10
    materials provided to Committee, 193
    misleading containers, 94
    prominence of required information,
        100 n.4, 101 n.7
Waxman, Henry A., 64
West Virginia requirements
    artificial colors, flavors, and
        preservatives, 130, 132
    cider products, 118 n.9, 130
    discrepancies between Federal require-
        ments and, 201
    honey, 119 n.10
    materials provided to Committee, 193
    prominence of required information,
        100 n.5
White House Conference on Food,
        Nutrition, and Health, 3, 51,
        66, 109
Wholesome Meat Act, 48
Wholesome Poultry Products Act, 48
Wild rice, 11, 14, 21, 125-126, 197, 201, 208
Wiley, Harvey, 39, 41
Wilms, Heinz, 148
Wisconsin requirements
    artificial colors, flavors, and
        preservatives, 130 n.12
    discrepancies between Federal require-
        ments and, 201
    materials provided to Committee, 194
    prominence of required information,
        99 n.1, 101 n.7

Wisconsin requirements, *continued*
    wild rice, 125
Wyoming requirements
    discrepancies between Federal require-
        ments and, 201
    honey, 119 n.10
    materials provided to Committee, 194

Young, Frank E., 147